Sarra Ben Rejeb
Jasser Yaacoubi

Tumor budding in primary pancreatic adenocarcinoma

Sarra Ben Rejeb
Jasser Yaacoubi

Tumor budding in primary pancreatic adenocarcinoma

Analysis on digital images

ScienciaScripts

Imprint

Cover image: www.ingimage.com

This book is a translation from the original published under ISBN 978-613-9-52530-0.

Publisher:
Sciencia Scripts
is a trademark of
Dodo Books Indian Ocean Ltd. and OmniScriptum S.R.L publishing group

120 High Road, East Finchley, London, N2 9ED, United Kingdom
Str. Armeneasca 28/1, office 1, Chisinau MD-2012, Republic of Moldova, Europe
Managing Directors: Ieva Konstantinova, Victoria Ursu
info@omniscriptum.com

Printed at: see last page
ISBN: 978-620-8-63463-6

TABLE OF CONTENTS

INTRODUCTION

Pancreatic cancer is the 10th most common cancer and the 7th leading cause of cancer death worldwide [1].

Histologically, ductal adenocarcinoma represents 90% of malignant tumors of the pancreas and is characterized by a poor prognosis due to often late diagnosis with an overall 5-year survival rate, all stages combined, not exceeding 10% [2].

Early-stage surgery is the only potentially curable alternative. However, even with complete cancer surgery (R0), tumor recurrence is observed in approximately 70 to 90% of cases within two years [3,4]. Thus, resectability remains the determining factor in the management of pancreatic cancer.

However, many other histological parameters condition the prognosis; among them: histological type, histological grade, vascular emboli, perineural sheathing, locoregional extension, lymph node involvement and the quality of surgical excision. These parameters are currently well recognized as independent prognostic factors predictive of tumor aggressiveness, local recurrence and distant metastases [5].

However, these criteria now appear insufficient to predict the evolution of pancreatic cancer since most patients with pancreatic cancer develop local recurrence after surgery or therapeutic resistance.

In this context, the identification of the pathophysiological mechanisms involved in tumor aggressiveness has become a major challenge. Among these histological criteria, the phenomenon of epithelial-mesenchymal transition (EMT) seems to be associated with tumor aggressiveness and chemoresistance of carcinomas through acquisitions, at the level of carcinoma cells, of mesenchymal properties conferring on these cells a power of invasion and distant extension [6].

From anatomopathological point of view, it is currently well established that tumor budding (TB) is an independent histo-prognostic factor whose histological translation is determined by tumor budding in the form of isolated cells or clusters of less than 5 cells [7].

Since its first description in 1960, tumor budding has benefited as a new histo-prognostic factor through numerous studies [6,8]. Indeed, in colorectal cancers, BT is a predictive factor of lymphatic emboli, lymph node metastases, recurrence and death at 5 years regardless of the stage [9,10].

However, in pancreatic cancer, although the prognostic impact of BT has been suggested through numerous studies [6,8], this histological parameter is not yet systematically taken into consideration in current practice probably due to the absence of precise recommendations regarding the methodology and quantification systems on the one hand and a relatively difficult, time-consuming and poorly reproducible calculation on standard histological sections on the other hand.

It is in this context that the use of artificial intelligence (AI) applied to pathological anatomy constitutes a promising alternative.

Hence the interest of this work, the objectives of which were:

- Calculating the tumor Budding score in pancreatic adenocarcinomas by artificial intelligence.
- To analyze its prognostic value by correlation with clinical and histological parameters, overall survival and event-free survival.

METHODS

1. Presentation of the work:

This is a descriptive, cross-sectional, bicentric study. on cases of primary adenocarcinoma of the pancreas, collected from the pathological anatomy and cytology departments of the Internal Security Forces Hospital of La Marsa and the Charles Nicolle Hospital over a period of 14 years, i.e. between 2008-2022. Our material was of interest to:

- Pancreatic and liver biopsies
- Surgical parts (cephalic pancreatectomy, caudal pancreatectomy)

2. Population studied:

2.1. Inclusion criteria:

We included in this study all patients with primary adenocarcinoma of the pancreas diagnosed on surgical specimen , pancreatic or liver biopsy diagnosed in the Pathological Anatomy and Cytology department of the FSI and HCN Hospital during the study period.

2.2. Non-inclusion criteria:

Not included in this study:

- Patients with intraductal papillary mucinous tumor without a focus of invasion.
- Other histological types (neuroendocrine or mesenchymal tumors).
- Patients with ampullary, gallbladder or biliary tract adenocarcinoma.

2.3. Exclusion criteria:

We excluded from our study:

- Patients whose clinical records were unusable.
- The biopsy samples are small and not very representative.
- Biopsy samples whose technical quality was not optimal having generated artifacts during the digitalization of the images.

3. Collection of clinical data:

We selected cases from the computerized database of the Marsa Internal Security Forces Hospital and the Department of Pathology of Charles Nicolle Hospital. The keywords used were: *adenocarcinoma/carcinoma/pancreas.* Epidemiological and clinical data were collected from the medical records of patients from the General Surgery Department of the Marsa Internal Security Forces Hospital and the A21 General Surgery Department of Charles Nicolle Hospital.

These data concerned: age, sex, medical and surgical history, clinical warning signs, clinical examination data, radiological examinations requested, therapeutic indication, type of surgery, post-operative complications.

4. Collection of anatomo-pathological data:

We collected pathological data from pathological reports. These data included:

- Tumor size for surgical specimens
- Histological type and subtype according to the 2019 "World Health Organization" classification (Appendix 1)
- Histological grade
- Perineural sheaths: present/absent
- Vascular emboli: present/absent

- The stage (pT) and the lymph node status (pN) according to the pTumor-Node-Metastases (pTNM) classification of the "American Joint Committee on Cancer" in its 8th edition of 2017 (Appendix 2)

- Resection quality (margins: section slice and retroportal blade): positive/negative

5. Collection of evolving data:

We collected the following evolutionary data:

- Overall survival
- The recidivism
- The appearance of metastases

6. Tumor budding study:

6.1. Morphological study:

Given the lack of specific recommendations applicable to pancreatic cancer, the study of BT was performed according to the recommendations established at the 2016 BT international consensus conference for colon cancer [11]. BT was defined by the presence of isolated tumor cells or clusters of <5 cells.

For each case, a review of all slides containing tumor material stained ~~with~~ hematoxylin and eosin (HE) was performed by two pathologists in order to select areas of high BT ("hot-spot"), at the level of the tumor invasion front or intra-tumorally.

For each selected blade, the BT was evaluated morphologically by two pathologists on the multi-head microscope (NIKON Eclipse Ni-U) at x 20 magnification, corresponding to a field diameter of 0.785mm2.

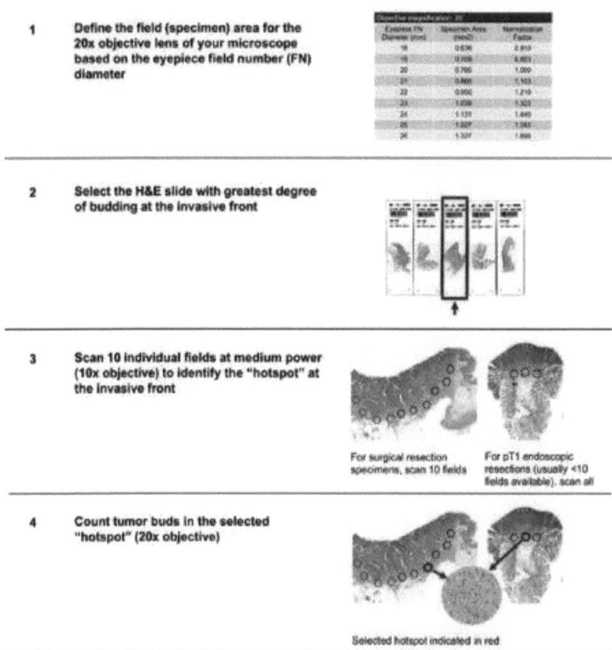

Figure 1: ITBCC recommendations for calculating tumor budding[11]

6.2. Study by artificial intelligence:

We subsequently calculated the BT by a semi-automated approach using AI using QUPATH software (version 0.2.1) [12] open access allowing the analysis of high-resolution digital images of microscopic sections.

Most published studies that used AI for the study of BT performed the analysis on DAB immunohistochemical staining images (using the anti-CK antibody).

By typing the keywords: QUPATH and BT on the PUBMED search engine, two publications were found, only one of which used the QUPATH software for the analysis of BT on sections stained with HE in intrahepatic cholangiocarcinomas [13] .

We therefore used the same methodological approach in this work.

For each case, the territories selected for the calculation of BT by morphological method were examined at x 10 magnification and then digitized using the NIS digital imaging software connected to the NIKON microscope (Figure 2). These images were previously saved in high-resolution GIF format (300 dpi).

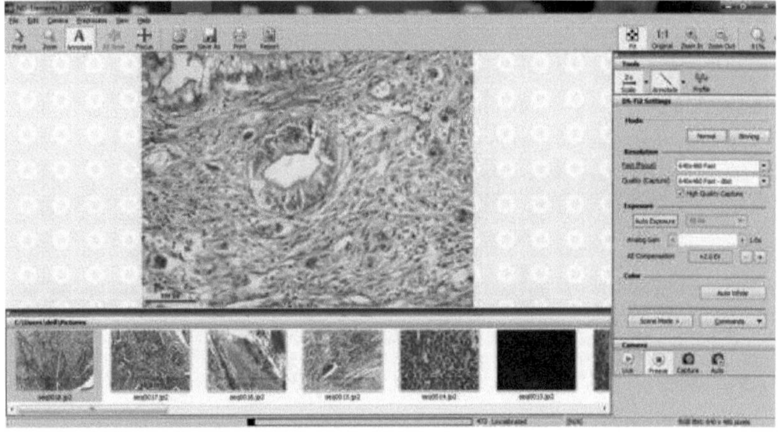

Figure 2: Image of a microscopic section on the NIS software

Subsequently, the scanned images were uploaded to the QUPATH software. An annotation was performed in order to segment the image according to the criteria: tumor (Red), stroma or lymphocytes (in yellow) subsequently allowing the detection of tumor cells (Figure 3).

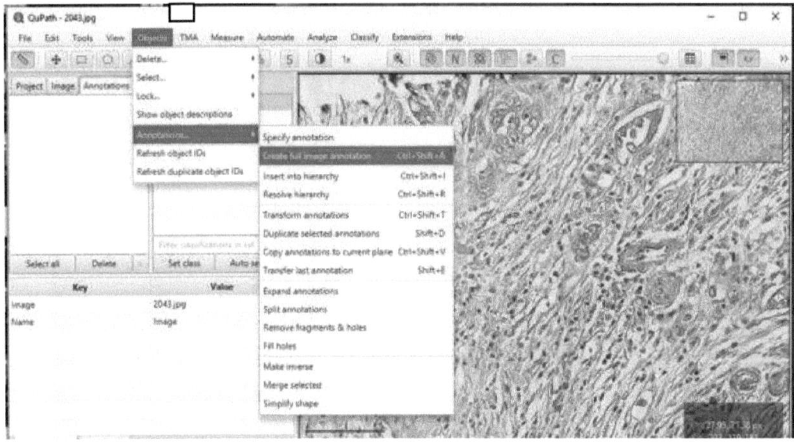

Figure 3: Creating an image annotation on QUPATH software

We used the "cell detection" functionality which allows easy detection of isolated tumor cells or small cell groups compared to tumor clusters and masses and thus their manual count on the software.

On each digitized image at x10 magnification, we defined 5 rectangles. Each rectangle corresponded to a surface area of 0.785mm2 taking into account the "hot spot" areas. Within each rectangle, we used the "cell-detection" functionality which allowed us to surround the tumor cells taking into account the characteristics of the nucleus and the pixel difference for a sigma of the nucleus defined between 3 and 8 pixels (Figure 4).

The total BT score corresponded to the average of the 5 rectangles (i.e. 5 fields with a surface area of 0.785mm2).

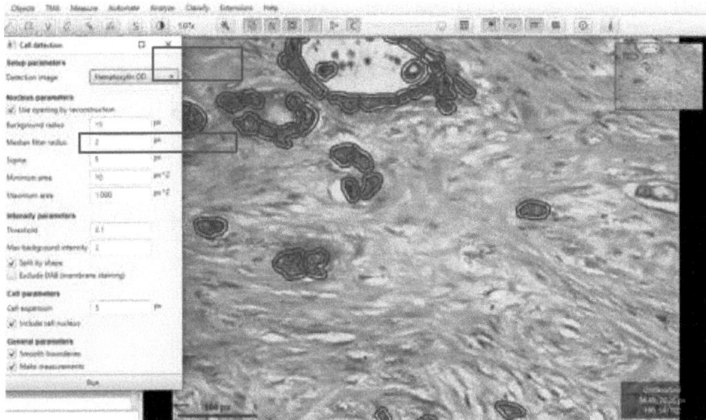

Figure 4: Detection of isolated or small group tumor cells on QUPATH software

For some cases, false positives were detected (myofibroblastic cells of the stroma or remnants of neuroendocrine islets), it was possible to correct them by deselecting them (in yellow) (Figure 4).

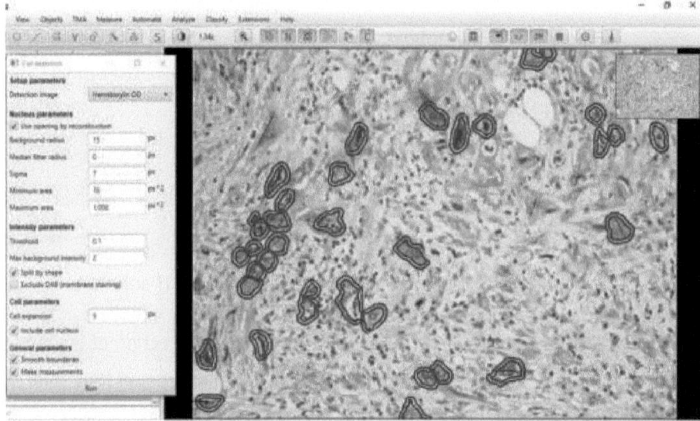

Figure 5: Identification of false positives on the QUPATH software

The final BT count was then easily carried out for each case.

6.3. Classification of tumor budding:

For each calculation method (morphological/digitalized), the calculated BT was categorized into 3 groups according to the ITBCC recommendations:

- ✓ **BUD1:** 0 -4 buds
- ✓ **BUD2:** 5-10 buds
- ✓ **BUD3 :>** 10 buds

☐The final BT score was divided into two groups:

- ➢ **Low:** BUD1
- ➢ **Raised:** BUD2-BUD3

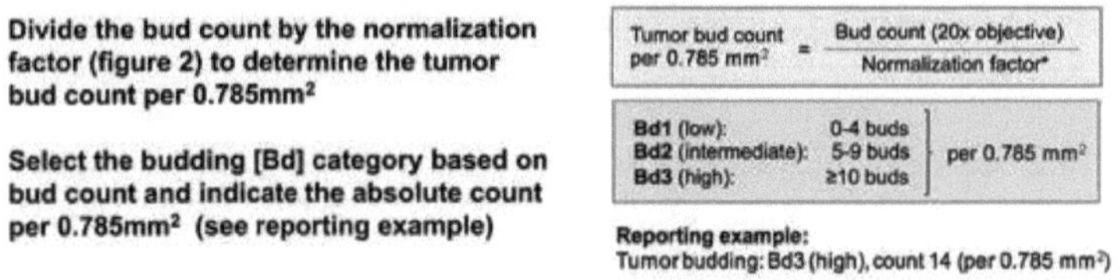

Divide the bud count by the normalization factor (figure 2) to determine the tumor bud count per 0.785mm²

Select the budding [Bd] category based on bud count and indicate the absolute count per 0.785mm² (see reporting example)

Tumor bud count per 0.785 mm² = Bud count (20x objective) / Normalization factor*

Bd1 (low): 0-4 buds
Bd2 (intermediate): 5-9 buds
Bd3 (high): ≥10 buds
per 0.785 mm²

Reporting example:
Tumor budding: Bd3 (high), count 14 (per 0.785 mm²)

Figure 6: ITBCC recommendations for the classification of tumor budding [11]

7. Statistical study:

Statistical analysis was performed using SPSS 21 software. Comparison of means was performed using the *Mann – Whitney U test*.

Comparisons of percentages and search for associations were performed by Pearson's chi-square test, and by Fisher's two-tailed exact test.

The prognostic factors studied were: age, sex, tumor size, histological subtype, stage, vascular emboli, perineural sheathing, quality of excision, lymph node status, recurrences, distant metastases and mortality.

Survival data were studied by establishing survival curves according to the Kaplan Meier method and compared by the Log rank test in univariate analysis.

RESULTS

1. Descriptive study:

Among the 37 cases previously collected, 25 cases met our inclusion and exclusion criteria (i.e. 12 cases excluded: eight patients were lost to follow-up and four patients whose samples were unusable).

1.1. Age :

The mean age of the participants was 62 ± 10 years. The distribution of patients by age group is summarized in **Figure 7.**

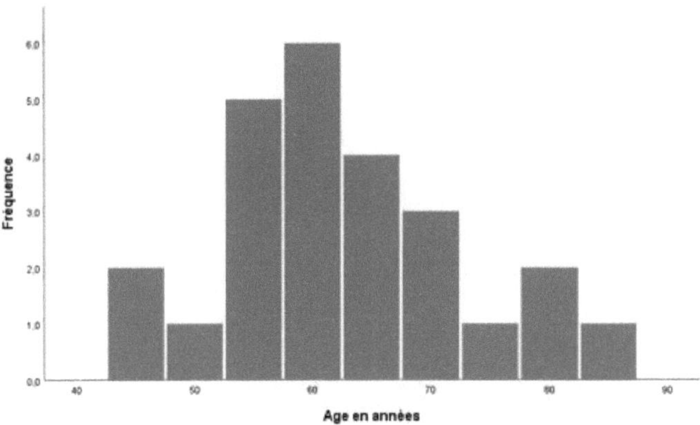

Figure 7: Distribution of patients by age

1.2. Gender:

The male/female ratio was 2.57 (**Figure 8**)

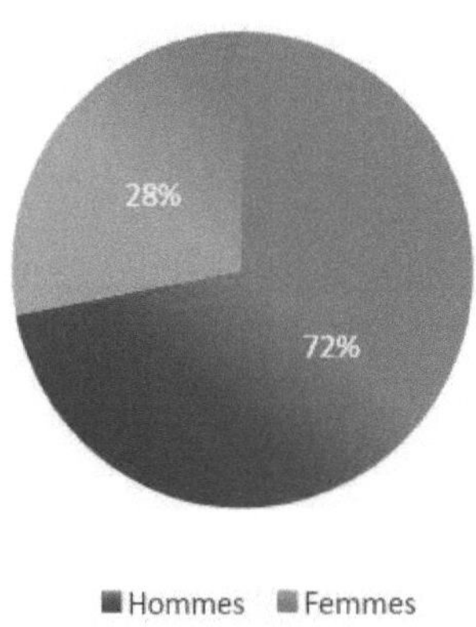

Figure 8: Distribution of patients by gender

1.3. Habits:

Alcohol consumption was found in 36% of our patients.

Smoking was found in 56% of our patients.

We have summarized these results in Figure 9.

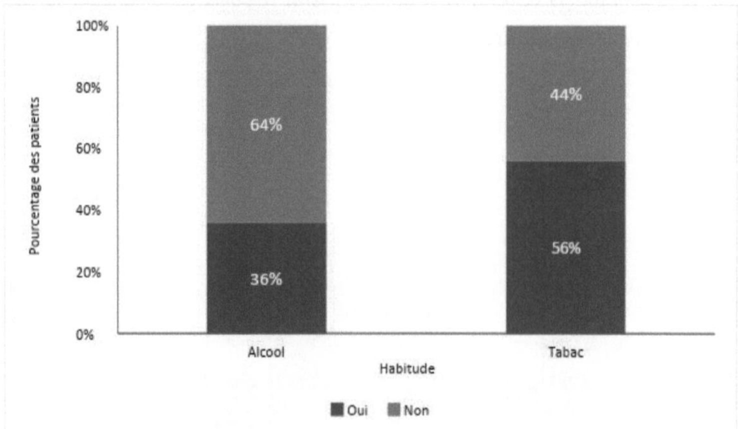

Figure 9: Distribution of patients according to their habits

1.4. Circumstances of discovery:

The warning signs found in our patients were: abdominal pain in 96% of cases, deterioration of general condition in 8% of cases, jaundice in 72% of cases and dark urine in 64% of cases. The minimum consultation time was 2 weeks in 68% of cases, among which 52% after at least one month.

1.5. Imaging data:

The mean diameter of the common bile duct (CBD) was 14.52 ± 5 mm.

The mean diameter of the Wirsung was 4.56 ± 2 mm. The pancreatic tumor was located in the head in 20 patients (80% of cases).

The remaining CT scan findings at the time of initial diagnosis are shown in **Figure 10.**

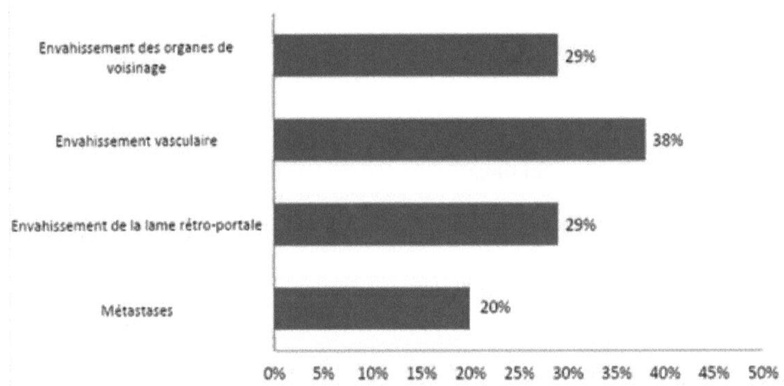

Figure 10: Results of our patients' CT scan data

1.6. Therapeutic decisions:

Surgery was performed in 20 patients (80% of cases). The type of intervention is reported in **Figure 11.**

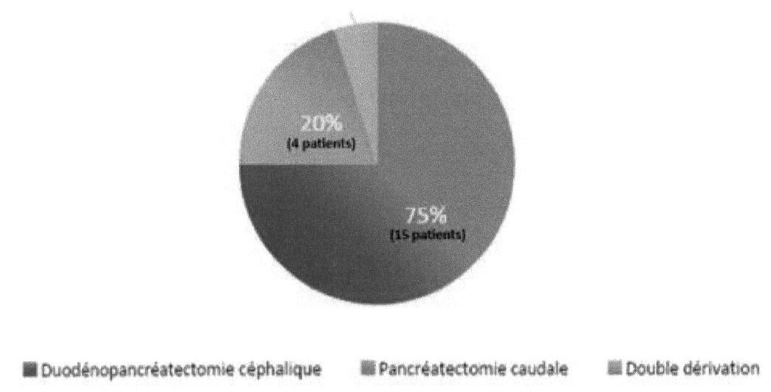

Figure 11: Distribution of the different surgical techniques used in the 20 patients operated on for pancreatic adenocarcinoma

Other therapeutic modalities are summarized in **Table I.**

Table I: The main therapeutic modalities other than surgery in the 25 patients with pancreatic adenocarcinoma

Treatment	Effective
Induction treatment	3
Adjuvant treatment	14
Prosthesis	8

1.7. Anatomopathological data:

1.7.1. Type of samples.

The samples were of the following type:

- Biopsies in 6 cases
- Surgical parts in 19 cases, divided into:
  - ➔ DPC parts (15 cases)
  - ➔ SPG Parts (4 cases)

1.7.2. Macroscopic data.

Macroscopic data were available for all 19 operated patients. The mean tumor size was 33.2 ± 13 mm

The tumor was located cephalically in 15 cases and caudally in 4 cases.

Macroscopic invasion of the retroportal lamina was observed in 3 cases.

A macroscopic extension to neighboring organs in 2 cases.

1.7.3. Microscopic data.

The histological type was adenocarcinoma in all cases (WHO classification 2019 annex 1).

The anatomopathological data are summarized in **Table II.**

Table II: Results of the anatomopathological study of our series

			Number
Histological subtypes		**Conventional Ductal**	24
		Adenosquamous	1
Histological grades		**G1-G2**	18
		G3	7
Perineural sheathing		**Yes**	20
		No	5
Vascular emboli		**Yes**	13
		No	12
Limits of resection (on surgical specimen)		**Invaded**	4
		Healthy	15
pTN classification (on surgical specimen)	**T**	**T1**	1
		T2	9
		T3	8
		T4	1
	N	**N0**	8
		N1	9
		N2	2

1.8. Tumor Budding Study:

1.8.1. Study by morphological method:

A BT tumor budding (>0 buds) was observed in all cases (**100%**). It was high (BUB2-BUD3) in **48% of cases** . The distribution of patients according to the morphological Budding score is summarized in **Table III** .

Table III: Distribution of patients according to the morphological Budding score

Budding	Effective	Percentage
BUD 1 (0 – 4 buds)	13	52
BUD 2 (5 – 9 buds)	4	16
BUD 3 (≥ 10 buds)	8	32
Total	25	100

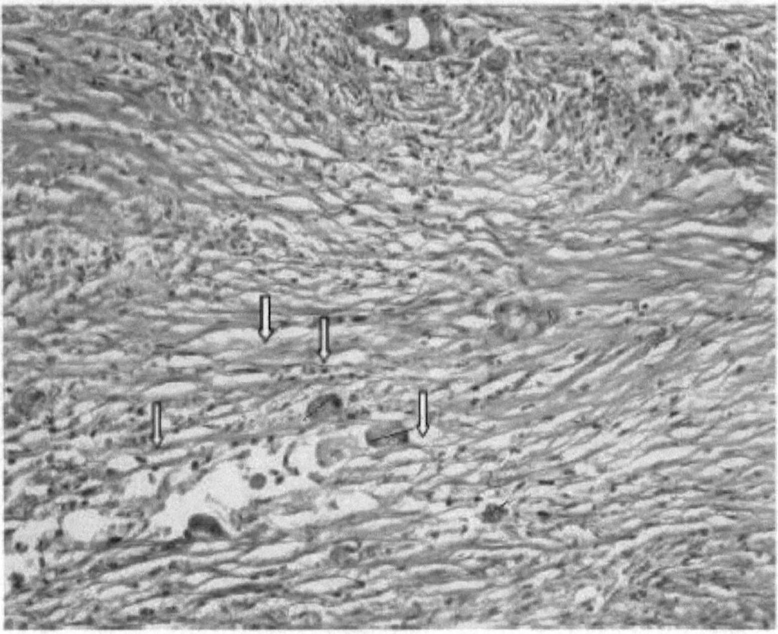

Figure 12: Ductal adenocarcinoma with presence of tumor budding classified as BUD1 (Hematoxylin Eosin X 20)

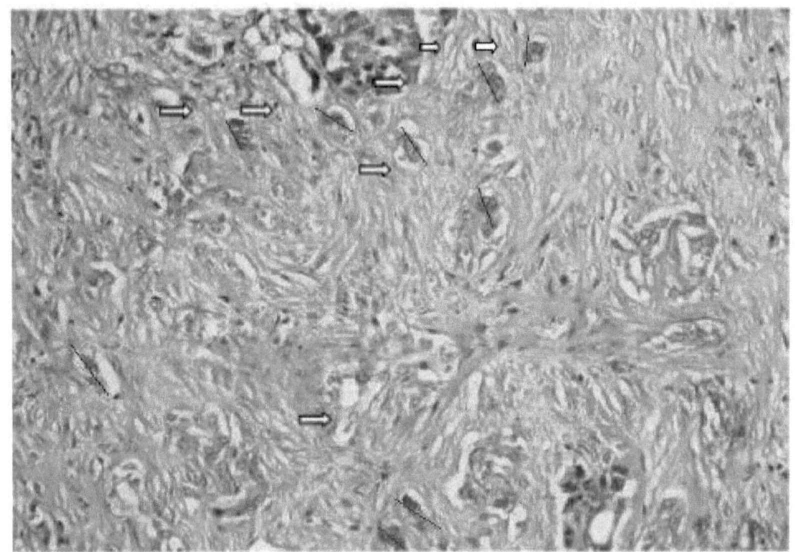

Figure 13: Ductal adenocarcinoma with presence of tumor budding classified as BUD2 (Hematoxylin Eosin X 20)

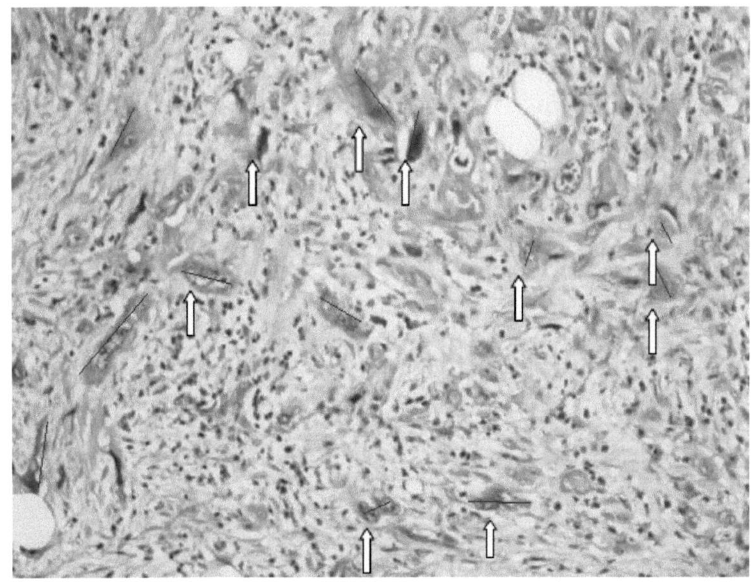

Figure 14: Ductal adenocarcinoma with presence of tumor budding classified as BUD3 (Hematoxylin Eosin X 20)

1.8.2. Study by QUPATH software:

A BT tumor budding (>0buds) was found in **80%** of cases. It was elevated in 56% of patients. We have summarized these results in **Table IV** .

Table IV: Distribution of patients according to the Budding score by artificial intelligence

Budding	Effective	Percentage
BUD 1 (0 – 4 buds)	11	44
BUD 2 (5 – 9 buds)	11	44
BUD 3 (≥ 10 buds)	3	12
Total	25	100

1.9. Evolutionary data:

1.9.1. Post-operative complications:

They occurred in 60% of operated patients. They were non-specific in 55% of cases and specific in 45% of cases (digestive hemorrhage in 25% of cases, pancreatic fistula in 20% of cases).

1.9.2. Prediction:

Locoregional recurrence was observed in 37% of cases (mean time of 170 days). Distant metastases had appeared in 37% of cases (mean time of 141 days). For an average follow-up period of 18 months, death occurred in 72% of cases.

2. Analytical study:

2.1. Comparison of Budding by Morphological Method/Artificial Intelligence

The number of buds by the morphological method varied between 1 and 37 with a mean of 8, a median of 4 and a standard deviation of 8.

The number of buds by the semi-automated method ranged from 0 to 19 with a mean of 6, a median of 6 and a standard deviation of 5.

A reduction in the number of cases with a BT BUD3 score (>10) was observed using the semi-automated approach (32% by morphological approach versus 12% using QUPATH software).

The comparison between these two methods did not show any significant difference with a p=0.589. The sensitivity and specificity were 60%.

The positive predictive value was 50% and the negative predictive value was 69%.

2.2. Association of morphological tumor budding with clinical and histological parameters

A statistically significant association was found between high BT and age > 72 years (**p = 0.03**).

Eighty-five percent of common ductal tumors had a high Budding score **(p = 0.07)** .

Fifty-four percent of patients with advanced lymph node localization or pT stage had a high tumor Budding score, however this difference was not statistically significant (p=0.53 and **p=0.08**).

These results are summarized in Table V

Table V: Study of factors associated with tumor budding.

	Low morphological budding (n=12) (%)	Severe morphological budding (n=13) (%)	P
Age >72 years	0 (0)	4 (31)	**0.03**
Male gender	10 (83)	8 (62)	0.22
Tobacco	9 (75)	5 (36)	0.07
Jaundice	11 (61)	7 (39)	0.04
Pain	12 (100)	12 (92)	0.52
Tumor size	9 (75)	8 (62)	0.38
Conventional root canal subtype	6 (50)	11 (85)	**0.07**
Adenosquamous subtype	0 (0)	1 (8)	0.52
Limits of tumor resection	1 (8)	3 (23)	0.46
Presence of perineural sheathing	6 (50)	10 (77)	0.53
Presence of vascular embolus	3 (25)	8 (62)	0.20
Histological grade 3	1 (8)	4 (31)	0.61
T >2	6 (50)	4 (31)	**0.08**
Presence of N+ lymph node metastasis	4 (25)	7 (54)	0.53

2.3. Survival study

The parameters studied are: age, sex, tumor size, histological subtype, resection margins, perineural sheathing, vascular emboli, number of invaded lymph nodes, histological grade and BT.

2.3.1. Local recurrence

The overall cumulative local recurrence-free survival is represented by the following figure.

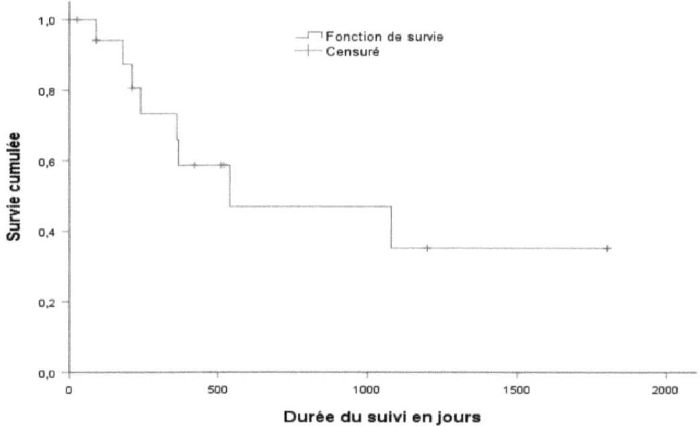

Figure 15: Overall cumulative local recurrence-free survival

Only the presence of perineural sheathing was a factor significantly associated with local recurrence with a p=0.031

This result is shown in the following figure.

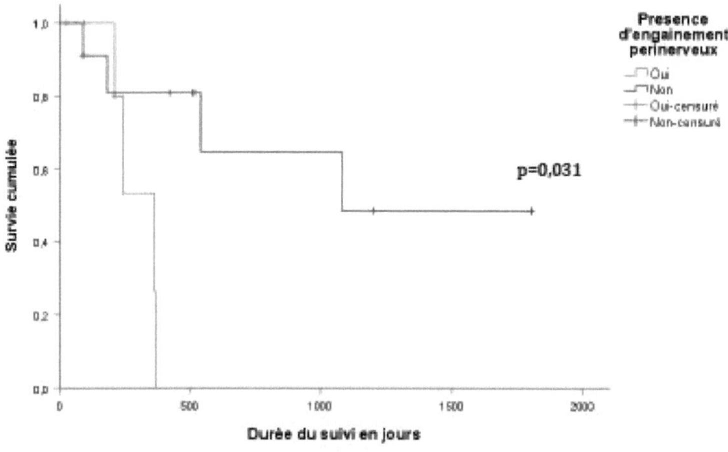

Figure 16: Curve of the development of the incidence of local recurrence according to perineural sheathing

2.3.2. Metastatic recurrence

The overall cumulative survival without metastatic recurrence is represented by the following figure.

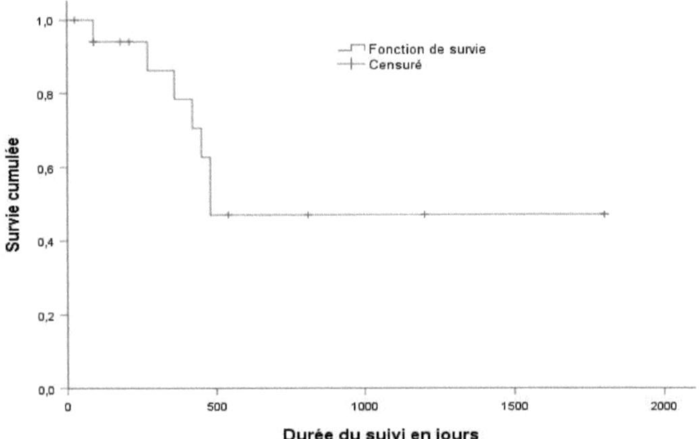

Figure 17: Overall cumulative survival without metastatic recurrence

The adenosquamous histological subtype, the presence of vascular emboli and the high histological grade were variables significantly associated with metastatic recurrence with p values of 0.001, 0.048 and 0.021 respectively.

These results are shown in the following 3 figures.

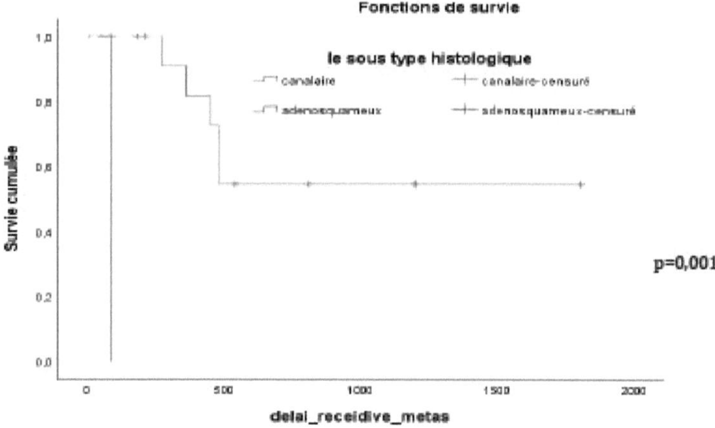

Figure 18: Curve of the development of the incidence of metastatic recurrence according to the histological subtype

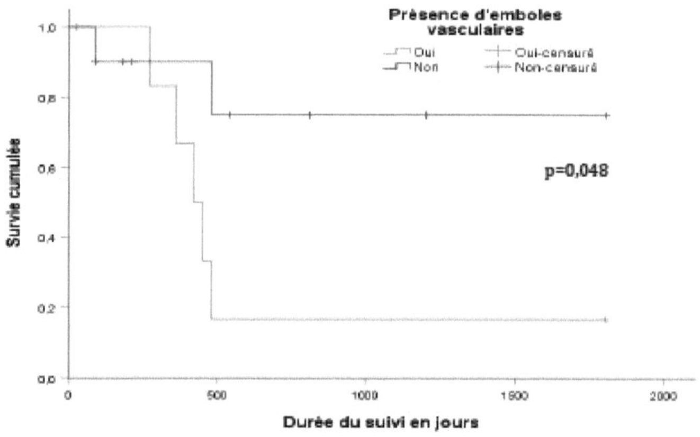

Figure 19: Curve of the development of the incidence of metastatic recurrence according to vascular emboli

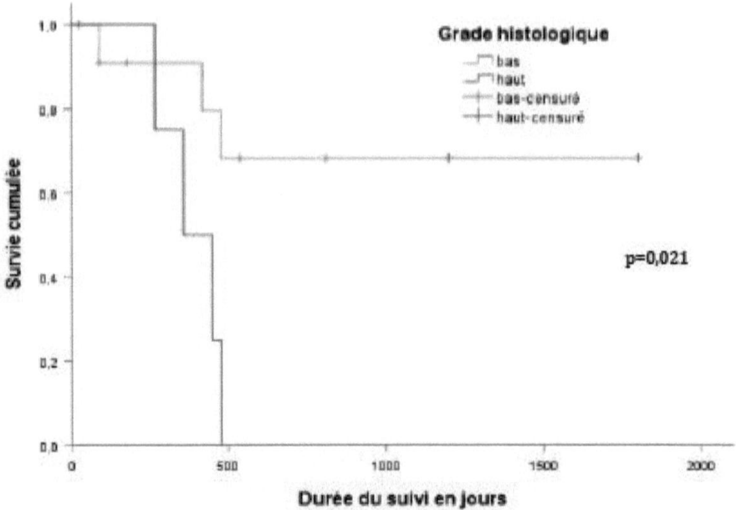

Figure 20: Curve of the development of the incidence of metastatic recurrence according to histological grade

2.3.3. Death :

Factors significantly associated with mortality were histological grade with p=0.044 and high BT with p=0.038.

These results are shown in Figures 21, 22 and 23.

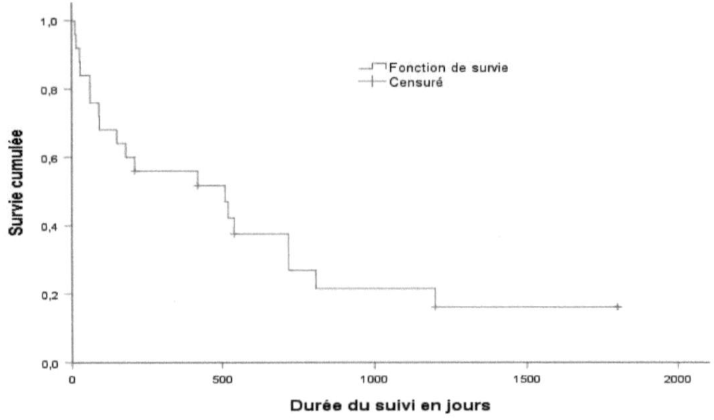

Figure 21: The overall survival curve

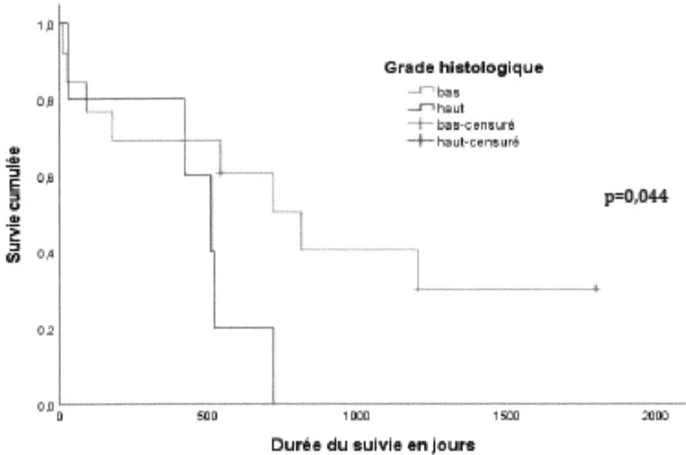

Figure 22: Death progression curve according to histological grade

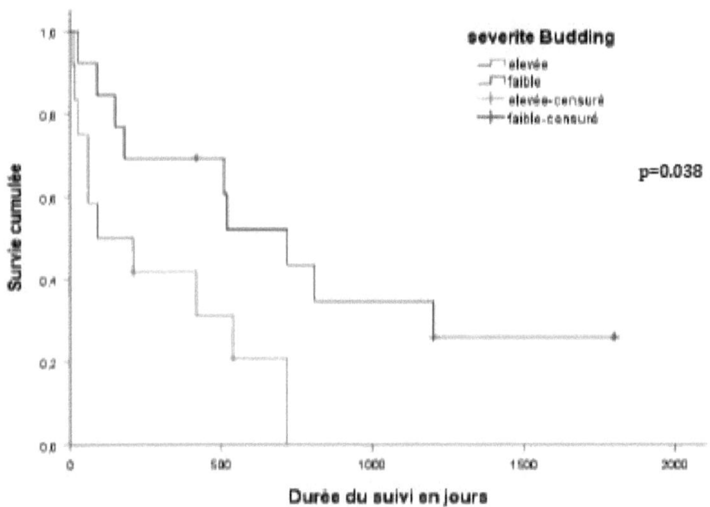

Figure 23: Death evolution curve according to tumor budding

DISCUSSION

1. Summary of the main results:

The descriptive study of the epidemiological characteristics of our patients with pancreatic cancer showed a mean age of **62 +/- 10 years and a male** predominance (72%).

Smoking was the predominant risk factor (56%).

The most common clinical signs were general condition deterioration (96%), abdominal pain (80%) and jaundice (72%).

From anatomopathological point of view the predominant histological subtype was **ductal carcinoma conventional (85%),** perineural sheathing was present in 80% of cases, vascular emboli were reported **in 55%** of cases.

Our study revealed the presence of tumor budding in **100%** of cases by morphological analysis and in **80% of cases** by approach using QUPATH artificial intelligence software

.

BT score was found in **56% of cases** by morphological method (**versus 48%** by QUPATH software)

The use of the semi- automated method allowed a reduction in the percentage of BUD3 category cases (from 32% to 12%).

Comparative analysis of the two methods did not reveal any statistically significant difference (p=0.589)

In univariate analysis, a statistically significant association was found between a high BT score and advanced age **(p=0.03) .**

In survival study: Tumor grade and BT significantly affected overall survival **(p=0.044, p=0.038 respectively).**

2. Strengths and limitations:

The main limitations of our study:

- The small sample size after application of the inclusion and exclusion criteria (unusable data, lost to follow-up, poor quality samples). However, it should be remembered that pancreatic cancer is rare and that the majority of similar studies have used a small number of cases (less than fifty)

- Retrospective data collection.

- The digitization of HE section images was performed using NIS software, which only allows fields previously defined under the microscope to be taken. Therefore, in our study, for good reproducibility and comparability of the two methods used, the hot spot territories chosen by screening the slide at low magnification and on which we calculated the BT morphologically were digitized on NIS software to extract them with QUPATH software.

However, our study has some strengths:

- To our knowledge, this is the first nationwide study to analyze the prognostic value of BT in pancreatic cancer using two approaches: conventional on HE section and semi-automated using QUPATH artificial intelligence software.

- Similarly, to our knowledge, this is the first national study to have used AI applied to anatomopathological studies.

- The digitalized approach used in our study guarantees a high-resolution image (300dpi) with a precision in cell detection that easily distinguishes isolated tumor cells from groups of poorly differentiated cells and avoids false positives.

3. Anatomopathological study:

3.1. The study of Tumor Budding:

3.1.1. Tumor Budding Concept:

Tumor budding is a pattern of carcinoma invasion defined by the presence of isolated cells or clusters of less than 5 cells at the invasion front [14].

It was first described in 1960 by Alexandru Dan Grigore et al and has benefited as a new histo-prognostic factor through numerous studies [11]. BT is considered as the histological translation of the epithelial-mesenchymal transition phenomenon [11]. It is a process of transformation of an epithelial cell into a cell of mesenchymal phenotype by loss of polarity and intercellular junctions [15]. This phenomenon would notably involve the loss of expression of the surface protein E-cadherin, a membrane adhesion protein [16]. This phenomenon allows the cell to acquire capacities for mobility and local and distant invasion. The poor prognostic value of BT has been well demonstrated in colorectal cancer and its presence justifies adjuvant chemotherapy after surgical resection [9].

Indeed, BT is now a powerful predictive factor of lymphatic emboli, lymph node metastases, recurrence and death at 5 years in colorectal cancers [10,11].

Conversely, in pancreatic cancer, although its prognostic value is strongly suggested, BT analysis is not yet systematically performed and reported due to the absence of precise recommendations regarding the methodology and quantification systems on the one hand and the difficulty of its evaluation on standard histological sections on the other hand [17,18]. In this context, the use of AI analysis could constitute a promising alternative to evaluate BT in digestive cancers in general and in pancreatic cancer in particular. Therefore, in our study, we evaluated BT in a series of pancreatic adenocarcinoma by two methods: a morphological approach on HE sections and a semi-automated approach on digitalized images incorporated into the QUPATH AI software.

Indeed, it is crucial to calculate tumor budding initially by morphological method before resorting to artificial intelligence in order to establish a solid and precise reference base. Morphology, as a traditional and proven approach, allows the pathologist a global and simultaneous analysis of all histopathological characteristics. This step is therefore essential to evaluate the results, the precision and the relevance of artificial intelligence in this context.

3.1.2. Morphological approach:

Many approaches have been used for the calculation of BT based on semi-quantitative or quantitative evaluation with different thresholds, particularly concerning the number of microscopic fields examined [17–22]

In colon cancer, the assessment of BT was the subject of a consensus developed at the international BT consensus conference in 2016. This consensus made it possible to standardize the method of BT assessment in colorectal cancer and to include it in the anatomopathological report [11]. Since its validation in colon cancer, many studies have extrapolated this assessment method in other digestive cancers and in particular pancreatic cancers. Therefore, in this work, as is the case in the study published by Karamitopoulou. E et al [18] and given its level of evidence, tumor budding was assessed morphologically according to the ITBCC recommendations at a magnification of X20 for an area of 0.785 mm^2, at the invasion front or in the center of the tumor [7]. By this morphological approach of analysis on HE sections, our results demonstrated the presence of tumor budding **in 100%** of cases of pancreatic adenocarcinoma. Indeed, by applying the definitions of the said recommendations, isolated tumor cells or clusters of < 5 cells were observed in all cases. These results are consistent with previous publications on this subject indicating that tumor budding is present in approximately 85 to 100% of pancreatic adenocarcinoma samples [6,7]. Indeed, in a multicenter national study, Chouat E. et al, analyzed BT on a series of 50 cases of ductal adenocarcinomas of the pancreas and reported the presence of BT in 100% of cases [7]. Our results, like those described in the literature, suggest that **tumor budding, as is the case with perineural sheathing, is a relatively frequent or even constant phenomenon in pancreatic cancer, which could explain on the one hand its aggressiveness and on the other hand could have a high diagnostic value of pancreatic cancer on biopsy samples** . [7].

In our study, in accordance with the ITBCC recommendations, the BT score was subdivided into two broad categories: Low (BD1: 0-4 budds) and High (BD2: 5-10 budds, BD3: >10 budds). According to this conventional morphological approach, a high BT score was found **in 48% of cases** . Our results are similar to those published nationally by Chouat E et al, who reported a high BT in 50% of cases using the morphological method on HE sections and 56% using immunostaining with the anti-pan CK antibody [7]. However, the percentage of high BT in our series was slightly lower compared to the results of international studies where a high BT score was reported at a variable frequency of 56 to 80% of cases [5,7]. These differences can be partly explained by the differences in methodology for quantifying tumor budding, microscopic magnification, microscopic field diameter, the possible use of immunohistochemistry to identify tumor cells labeled by pan-CK as well as the use of AI software [13]. Conversely, in a study similar to ours, Sadozai H. et al analyzed the prognostic value of BT in pancreatic cancer in association with the immune microenvironment [23]. In a series of 111 cases of pancreatic ductal adenocarcinoma, the authors used the same BT subdivision criteria as in our study. They demonstrated the presence of a high BT in 48.6% of cases, which is consistent with our results [23]. **Therefore, a standardization of the evaluation method as well as BT classification criteria are necessary for better reproducibility and comparability of the results of the different studies.**

3.1.3. Analysis on QUPATH software:

Although the ITBCC consensus conference morphological approach is defined by simple histological criteria, it is relatively time-consuming and suffers from a lack of reproducibility among pathologists, which significantly limits its application in routine practice [16]. Similarly, the interpretation and recognition of tumor budding images on standard HE staining sections can be hampered by many histological parameters including an inflammatory stroma, the presence of mucin or tumor necrosis [16]. In this context, many alternatives have been proposed for the assessment of BT in colon cancer, including the use of immunolabeling of epithelial cells using an anti-CK antibody or the use of AI software applied to pathological anatomy [16]. Indeed, the analysis of tumor budding, a relatively difficult and time-consuming task for the pathologist, could be simplified by algorithms allowing the counting of tumor cells isolated on digital images [16,24]. The software developed for the assessment of BT is mostly based on the deep-machine learning technique, which is particularly effective in the field of image processing [16,25–30]. These algorithms have been developed for analysis either on a whole HE slide ("whole slide image") or on a previously defined area, in particular the invasion front. However, whatever the AI analysis functionalities used, the first parameter to decide before any image analysis is the support for said analysis. Therefore, in our study context, **the quality of the digitized images is an essential requirement for the reliability of the results of BT analysis by artificial intelligence** . Nowadays, the digitization of whole HE slides has become fast, precise and high resolution thanks to slide scanners capable of digitizing hundreds of slides per hour [31]. This digitization is based on a pyramidal scan of each area of the slide with different objectives with a definitive assembly allowing the development of a virtual slide [31]. However, given its high cost and in the event of the unavailability of a slide scanner, low-cost alternatives for digitizing HE slides have been proposed, including microscopic photography and assembly using suitable software [31]. In our study, given the unavailability of a slide scanner, we opted for the "store and forward" static imaging technique, the digitization of HE slides was therefore carried out by microscopic photography on the NIKON microscope connected to the NIS software. Thus, for a better comparability of the semi-automated approach to the morphological method in the evaluation of BT, we digitized the hot spot fields on which the calculation was previously performed on HE sections. These images were previously saved in high-resolution GIF format (300 dpi), which guarantees optimal image quality for analysis on AI software. Similarly, the analysis of the digitized images improves the contrast and color intensity, which makes it possible to catch up with any false negatives from the microscope analysis, particularly on sections with low staining [16].

Most of the studies that used AI for BT analysis used paid or limited access software [16]. In our study, we opted for the AI software applied to pathological anatomy QUPATH, which is open and free of charge and little known in Tunisia. Indeed, in reference to the methodology used by Budeau KL et al, we extrapolated the morphological quantification approach of ITBCC on optical microscopy to images on the QUPATH software [13]. This digital pathology software allows pathologists to obtain reproducible results in a short time in order to provide quality data, particularly for the analysis of large series. Similarly, it is open and free of charge software, which constitutes an opportunity for pathologists in countries with a low socio-economic level to learn about AI applied to pathological anatomy at low cost [32]. The fundamental principle of analysis on the QUPATH software is the possibility of segmenting or annotating the incorporated image into: tumor cells, stroma and inflammatory elements. Therefore, thanks to its "cell detection" functionality, the QUPATH software allows the distinction of isolated tumor cells from poorly differentiated cell groups with great specificity. The algorithm of this software is based in this context on the characteristics of the nucleus, namely: the shape, size and pixel difference between the nucleus and the cytoplasm for a sigma of the nucleus defined between 3 and 8 pixels.

In our study, BT was observed in **80% of cases** using the semi-automated digital approach. Similarly, a high BT score was found in **56% of cases** using the QUPATH software (versus 48% by morphological approach), suggesting a greater precision of analysis by digital approach. However, it was noted that the use of the semi-automated method significantly reduced the number of Category BUD3 cases from 8 by conventional method to 3 on the QUPATH software **, suggesting a reduction in false positives compared to morphological analysis.** However, overall, there was no statistically significant difference between these two approaches (p = 0.589). Thus, the QUPATH software could be an interesting, fast and precise alternative for pathologists, **which would considerably reduce working time and facilitate the assessment of tumor budding** on samples of ductal adenocarcinoma of the pancreas or even the colon [13]. This would be even more advantageous by using a slide scanner which would allow on the one hand to analyze the entire slide and on the other hand to postpone the initial morphological analysis.

Furthermore, compared to the morphological evaluation method, the semi-automated approach using the QUPATH software seems more objective, reproducible and has the advantage of allowing a re-evaluation of the BT at any time even by other pathologists since the images are archived and can be consulted at any time on the software by other participants [13]. Similarly, it is possible to add new specific extensions to this software in order to add new functionalities, in particular an associated study of the inflammatory microenvironment.

3.1.4. Prognostic value of tumor budding:

According to the ITBCC recommendations, the tumor budding score is categorized into three levels for risk stratification [11,13]. In this study, with reference to the grading system published by Tanaka et al [33], we distinguished 3 groups BUD1-BUD2 and BUD3. Subsequently, we grouped into low BUD and high BUD. In our study, a statistically significant association was found between a high BT score and an advanced age of more than 72 years ($p = 0.03$). Similarly, these cases were mainly of common ductal subtype ($p = 0.07$) and advanced stage pT>pT2 ($p = 0.08$). These results are in agreement with previous publications on this subject having demonstrated a poor prognostic value of BT in pancreatic ductal adenocarcinoma. Indeed, in their publication O'Connor et al [34] demonstrated a statistically significant association between a high BT score (>10/10CFG) and histo-prognostic factors: grade, vascular and perineural invasion. Similarly, in our study, 54% of advanced stage patients (N+ and/or pT>pT2) and 77% of cases with perineural invasion had a high BT score. However, these results were not statistically significant ($p=0.53$; $p=0.32$ and $p=0.53$), which could be partly related to the small sample size.

It should be noted, however, that the majority of similar publications, such as our study, have not demonstrated a statistically significant relationship between BT and conventional histo-prognostic factors [5,7,8,35].

Conversely, in this study, a statistically significant association was found between tumor budding and overall survival (**p = 0.038**). These results, as reported in many studies, confirm the potential prognostic value of BT in pancreatic adenocarcinoma [5,7,34,36]. Moreover, in a meta-analysis published in 2019, Lawler et al demonstrated that patients with pancreatic adenocarcinoma with a high tumor budding score had a higher all-cause mortality rate compared to those with a low tumor budding score (HR 2.65, 95% CI 1.79–3.91, $P < 0.0001$) [37].

These results, although promising and converging towards an unfavorable prognostic value of tumor budding in pancreatic cancer, require a standardization of methods, particularly for the evaluation of the BT score, in order to establish precise and reproducible recommendations to introduce this factor into current practice in the anatomopathological study of pancreatic ductal adenocarcinomas. Indeed, some authors have only taken into consideration in their analysis the TB at the invasion front [5]. However, it is now well demonstrated that tumor budding has the same prognostic value both at the invasion front and at the center of the tumor [11,13]. On the other hand, some authors have suggested that the evaluation of tumor budding could be more precise and more reproducible using immunostaining of tumor cells with anti-CK antibodies [38]. Conversely, in a multicenter study, Hacking S et al [24] demonstrated that although immunohistochemical staining facilitates the detection of tumor cells, it has an intra- and inter-observatory reproducibility comparable to the morphological approach on HE slides. Finally, in the AI era, the use of digital pathology for BT assessment is a promising alternative that could significantly reduce the examination time and offer better accuracy and reproducibility. In this context, many studies have demonstrated a high diagnostic concordance (90-99%) between digital pathology through many software available on the market and the conventional morphological approach [39,40]. Many digital pathology imaging software have been developed, but access to these platforms remains difficult for some pathologists due to limited material and logistical resources. In this context, the QUPATH software as demonstrated through our study is an alternative of choice, freely accessible and relatively easy to handle, which allows pathologists, particularly in our country, to learn AI applied to pathological anatomy at the lowest cost. **However, it is necessary to establish, through multicenter studies, a consensus on the method of evaluating BT on the QUPATH software in order to definitively integrate it into current practice.**

3.1.5. Therapeutic implications:

In addition to its prognostic value, BT, as a marker of aggressiveness, could be used to guide treatment choice and predict therapeutic response. Indeed, patients with high BT could benefit from a more aggressive therapeutic approach, such as intensive adjuvant chemotherapy or specific targeted therapy. This approach has already been included in the treatment guidelines for stage II colon cancer. Indeed, the presence of high BT is now an indication for adjuvant chemotherapy according to the ESMO recommendations [41]. Similarly, some studies suggest that the presence of BT on biopsy specimens of rectal cancer is a factor of aggressiveness and could alone indicate neoadjuvant chemotherapy [42].

Unlike the situation for stage II colon cancer, in which the presence of a high BT could contribute to the therapeutic decision, BT in pancreatic cancer has not yet had an effective impact in current practice on adjuvant treatment decisions. Indeed, in pancreatic ductal adenocarcinoma, due to its aggressiveness and inherently poor prognosis, adjuvant chemotherapy with either FOLFIRINOX (folinic acid, fluorouracil, irinotecan, and oxaliplatin) or gemcitabine combined with capecitabine is recommended for all patients after curative resection regardless of the status of histo-prognostic factors including BT [43,44]. However, for patients who cannot benefit from double or triple therapy, treatment with gemcitabine alone is a reasonable option. In a retrospective analysis of the CONKO-001 trial, designed to compare adjuvant gemcitabine with observation in patients with pancreatic adenocarcinoma who underwent complete tumor resection with curative intent, the presence of BT was associated with decreased overall survival, whether or not patients were treated with adjuvant gemcitabine [45].

While BT appears to have little or no impact on the indication for adjuvant chemotherapy in pancreatic cancer, it may have predictive value for response to possible immunotherapy. Indeed, according to some studies, some authors have demonstrated that epithelial-mesenchymal transition (EMT) in pancreatic cancer, a biological phenomenon expressed by BT in histology, occurs in the context of a tumor microenvironment that escapes the immune system [44,46]. These studies have highlighted links between high BT, certain inflammatory markers, and the expression of Programmed Death Ligand 1 (PD-L1) on tumor cells.

These findings could influence the therapeutic management of pancreatic cancer, particularly predicting the response to immunotherapy.

3.2. Other anatomopathological data:

3.2.1. Histological type:

From anatomopathological point of view, pancreatic tumors constitute a broad spectrum of neoplasias whose histological classification is based on differentiation: epithelial or non-epithelial and their biological behavior: benign, pre-cancerous or malignant. Epithelial tumors are classified into endocrine and exocrine pancreatic tumors depending on the cell of origin, the latter being by far the most frequent, accounting for 95% of pancreatic tumors [47].

Within the group of exocrine tumors, as is the case in our series, ductal adenocarcinoma is the most common histological type, representing 90% of solid tumors of the pancreas [47]. It is characterized by a carcinomatous proliferation made of tubular and glandular structures with excretobiliary differentiation. Other morphological aspects can be observed, in particular a contingent with clear cells, cribriform or gyriform, which could have a negative prognostic impact [48]. Most ductal adenocarcinomas of the pancreas are well or moderately differentiated, characterized by a predominance of the glandular contingent [49]. Ductal adenocarcinoma is characterized by an abundant fibrous desmoplastic inflammatory stroma rich in matrix proteins which seems to play a role in tumor aggressiveness [50]

3.2.2. Histological grade:

Histological grade is an independent histo-prognostic factor [47]. It is established based on the following criteria: glandular differentiation, mucosecretion, nuclear atypia and mitotic index. Three histological grades are therefore defined: grade 1 corresponding to a well-differentiated adenocarcinoma composed of >90% glandular structures, grade 2 corresponding to a moderately differentiated adenocarcinoma composed of 50 to 95% glandular structures and grade 3 corresponding to a poorly differentiated adenocarcinoma composed of <50% glandular structures. Based on this grading system, a correlation has been established between histological grade and overall survival [47]. In our study, 72% of cases were histologically low grade, which is generally consistent with the predominance of well-differentiated forms of ductal adenocarcinoma which is around 80% in the literature [49].

3.2.3. Histological subtypes:

Several histological subtypes have been described, some of which have molecular abnormalities similar to common ductal adenocarcinoma [49]. Among these subtypes: adenosquamous carcinoma, anaplastic carcinoma, undifferentiated carcinoma, osteoclastic giant cell carcinoma, micropapillary carcinoma, signet ring cell carcinoma [49]. In our series, 85% of cases were of common form and 5% were classified as adeno-squamous type. These results are in agreement with the literature data, in fact, adenosquamous carcinoma as defined in the WHO classification by the association of two contingents >=30% of an adenocarcinoma and a squamous cell carcinoma is rare, estimated at 1-4% [47]. At the molecular level, it has been reported that adenosquamous carcinoma is characterized by a basal-like genomic profile and a poor prognosis with a mean survival of 9 months [47]. Therefore, the presence of a squamous cell contingent is a poor prognostic parameter that should be systematically reported.

3.2.4. Vascular emboli and perineural ensheathments:

The presence of vascular emboli and perineural sheathing constitute additional histo-prognostic factors [47]. In our study, vascular emboli were found in 55% of cases and perineural sheathing in 80% of cases. Indeed, it has been reported that the frequency of perineural sheathing was highest in pancreatic cancer, described in 70 to 100% of cases and correlated with a poor prognosis and shorter survival [51]. Perineural sheathing is observed both intra-tumorally and peripancreatically where the nervous structures are particularly developed [52].

The presence of perineural sheathing is a major diagnostic argument in pancreatic cancer, particularly on biopsy samples allowing differential diagnosis with chronic pancreatitis. Similarly, as is the case in our study, the presence of perineural sheathing is significantly associated with local recurrence ($p = 0.031$) [53].

3.2.5. pTNM staging:

The extension of ductal adenocarcinoma occurs rapidly in the retroperitoneal tissue, in the regional lymphatic relays, then at a distance in the celiac and superior mesenteric relays and finally in the liver by hematogenous metastasis [47]. TNM staging (UICC, 2017) is a major prognostic parameter that determines management and survival. Histologically, the T classification is based on tumor size regardless of its extra-pancreatic extension and the number of invaded lymph nodes determines the N category. In our study, 95% of tumors were >2cm in size or stage pT>pT1, similarly in 55% of cases lymph node involvement was found. This is, overall, in agreement with the data in the literature through which it has been shown that cancer is readily diagnosed at an advanced stage [47]. Indeed, in a recent meta-analysis of 693 cases of pancreatic cancer and aimed at developing a new staging system, Liang.Y et al demonstrated that 77.6% of cases were stage pT>pT1 and in half of the cases lymph node invasion was found [54].

In this same context, it has been clearly demonstrated that tumor size was directly correlated with survival [47]. Indeed, according to the work published by Takashi C et al, survival was 30.6 months in patients whose tumor was <2cm and 20.5 months in patients whose tumor was >=2cm ($p<0.001$) [55]. Similarly, other authors have demonstrated that tumor size was significantly more correlated with survival than extra-pancreatic extension. Indeed, survival would be more prolonged in patients with a tumor limited to the pancreas of size <3cm than those with extra-pancreatic extension [47].

3.2.6. Quality of excision:

The quality of surgical excision is a determining prognostic factor in resectable pancreatic cancer [47]. Indeed, it has been clearly demonstrated that patients with invaded margins after surgical resection had a mean survival of less than one year, which is similar to the overall survival of non-operated pancreatic cancer [56].

In our study, four patients had microscopically invaded resection margins after surgery, particularly of the retroportal lamina. However, careful macroscopic examination and a codified sampling protocol are necessary for an adequate assessment of the surgical margins of pancreatic cancer. Therefore, close collaboration between surgeons and pathologists during the macroscopic examination of surgical resection specimens for pancreatic cancer is strongly recommended.

4. Epidemiological, clinical and radiological data of pancreatic cancer:

4.1. Age :

In our study, the mean age of patients was **62+/- 10 years** and 72% of our patients were >55 years old. This is in line with the literature data on the epidemiology of pancreatic cancer. Indeed, pancreatic cancer mainly affects subjects aged over 55 years. In a recent epidemiological study published by Hu JX et al in 2021, it was shown that 92.6% of cases occur after the age of 55 with a peak between 65 and 75 years and a median of 70 years [1]. In Tunisia, we do not have data on a national scale, however, according to data from the national cancer registry of northern Tunisia published in March 2021, the mean age of patients with pancreatic cancer is **61.6 years** [2], fully in line with our results. Other authors, however, have suggested an older age of diagnosis and have demonstrated that in the majority of cases, the diagnosis of pancreatic cancer is made between the seventh and eighth decade [1,2].

4.2. Gender :

In our series, we noted a clear male predominance with a male/female ratio of 2.57. This is in agreement with most published works reporting a predilection of pancreatic cancer for the male sex with a variable sex ratio of 1.1 to 2 [2,3]. In the United States, the incidence of pancreatic cancer was estimated at 31,950 in men and 28,480 in women in 2020, similarly the mortality rate is significantly higher in male patients [1]. In Tunisia, in accordance with these data, the incidence was estimated at 3.8 in men and 2.3 in women [57].

4.3. Habits:

In our study, 56% of patients were smokers, which is consistent with literature data. Indeed, in their meta-analysis, Iodice et al [58] demonstrated a cause-and-effect relationship between smoking and pancreatic cancer [58]. The relative risk increases by 1.74 with the number of cigarettes smoked per day and the duration of tobacco intoxication [58,59]. This risk becomes zero after 10 years of cessation [58]. While the cause-and-effect relationship between smoking and pancreatic cancer seems well established, the carcinogenic power of alcohol is not clearly elucidated. In our series, 36% of patients were alcohol consumers. However, according to some authors, the relative risk greater than 1 between alcohol consumption and pancreatic cancer only really exists in heavy alcohol consumers defined by a dose greater than 30 grams per day [60]. Similarly, according to some studies, a statistically significant association has been reported between excessive alcohol consumption (>3 drinks/day) and pancreatic cancer. This association is not clearly established in cases of light to moderate consumption [61] . On the other hand, alcohol consumption is the main cause of chronic pancreatitis which is an established risk factor for pancreatic cancer [62]. It is therefore necessary to raise awareness among patients about the established carcinogenic role of tobacco and the potential role of alcohol in pancreatic cancer.

4.4. Circumstances of discovery:

It is well established that pancreatic cancer evolves in a silent mode in the early stages and patients are generally asymptomatic [2,63]. The functional signs reported by patients are related to invasion of a neighboring organ or to distant metastases [64].

The main reasons for consultation in our study were in agreement with those described in the literature represented by abdominal pain, jaundice and deterioration of general condition.

The following table summarizes the percentages in the literature.

Table VI: Summary table of the main reasons for consultation in the literature

	Noel et al [65]	**Zhao et al [66]**	**Billami et al [67]**	**Our series**
Abdominal pain	78.9	84.3	68.3	96
Jaundice	54.6	69.7	82.3	72
AEG	97.3	74.9	64.9	80
Others	58.9	65	23.7	44

4.5. Imaging data:

In our series, the radiological assessment was performed by thoraco-abdominopelvic CT scan which allowed the localization of the cephalic tumor in 80% of cases, which is consistent with the data in the literature [68]. Indeed, the thoraco-abdominopelvic CT scan is the key examination for diagnosis but also locoregional staging in order to assess tumor resectability and to highlight possible hepatic or pulmonary metastases or to suspect carcinomatosis [66,67]. Similarly, it allows the search for anatomical variants, for example a right hepatic artery arising from the superior mesenteric artery or the presence of an arcuate ligament. However, it should be remembered first that abdominal ultrasound can be performed as a first-line procedure, particularly in cases of jaundice; in order to highlight any possible dilation of the intra and extra hepatic bile ducts, thus confirming the retentional nature of the jaundice. It can also visualize the tumor in the event of cephalic location and if the size is > 15 mm [69].

Hepatic MRI is of interest in positive diagnosis but also for the search for hepatic metastases. It is also of interest in cases where CT scanning is contraindicated [67,70].

Echoendoscopy is very effective for the assessment of tumors less than 3 cm in diameter and is superior to CT examination, whereas the opposite is true for large tumors and, above all, it allows an ultrasound-guided biopsy to be performed [69].

4.6. Therapeutic decision:

4.6.1. Surgery

Surgery is the only potentially curative therapeutic alternative for pancreatic cancer [63]. The resectability rate in pancreatic cancer is reported to be in the order of 15-30% [65,66]. In our series, 80% of patients underwent surgery, however in only 76% the surgery was curative.

The resectability criteria depend essentially on the locoregional extension, particularly vascular. They are codified according to the radiological classification of the National Comprehensive Cancer Network (NCCN) (**Appendix 2)** .

Several authors recommend a first coelioscopy in order to avoid sometimes unnecessary laparotomies [71]. On the other hand, the type of intervention depends on the tumor location. In our study, fifteen patients were operated on by cephalic duodenopancreatectomy (CPD). Indeed, CPD is the basic curative treatment for cephalic tumors which are by far the most frequent [63]. While four patients underwent a left splenopancreatectomy (LSP). Indeed, in the case of a corpo-caudal tumor, surgical treatment which consists of a LSP is much less carried out since these clinically silent tumors are in the majority of cases diagnosed late at a locally advanced or metastatic stage and are not operable [64].

In our series, one patient underwent a double diversion for a locally advanced tumor. This is a palliative procedure involving the performance of a biliary diversion associated or not with a digestive diversion [4] thus allowing patients to be fed and reducing jaundice. This procedure can be replaced by the placement of a biliary or duodenal prosthesis by endoscopic route, which allows the obstacle to be removed, improves the quality of life and nutritional status with a view to chemotherapy in non-operable subjects [72].

4.6.2. Chemotherapy

For chemotherapy, several protocols are used in pancreatic cancer that vary according to the goal: induction chemotherapy was done in 3 patients aiming to reduce the initially borderline tumor size with a view to later surgery or palliative chemotherapy for metastatic tumors. Several criteria are involved in the choice of protocol, including the TNM stage (Appendix 3), histological criteria and general condition [73].

As for adjuvant chemotherapy, it is almost systematic in patients operated on for pancreatic adenocarcinoma whatever the stage.

4.7. Post-operative evolution and prognosis:

4.7.1. Post-operative evolution

Pancreatic surgery is a source of significant morbidity despite advances in resuscitation. This morbidity depends on the type of surgery, the general condition of the patient and the type of complications. In our series, 60% of patients presented postoperative complications. This percentage is generally close to the data reported in the literature where the frequency of these complications varied from 20% to 52% depending on the studies [74,75].

In our study, non-specific complications were the most frequent, particularly pneumonia and wall abscess observed in 15% of patients respectively. This is in agreement with the literature data where the most commonly described non-specific complication in the literature is surgical site infection, ranging from 14 to 35% [76,77].

Conversely, complications specific to pancreatic surgery were observed in 45% of cases. They were dominated by digestive hemorrhage (25%) and pancreatic fistula (20%). These results are, overall, consistent with the literature data through which pancreatic fistula constitutes the most frequent complication of pancreatic surgery, estimated at a variable frequency of 5 to 30% and responsible for a high mortality rate [78]. Conversely, digestive hemorrhage observed in 25% of cases in our series is a rather rare complication estimated at 1 to 8% [79], it can be responsible for 38% of mortality according to some authors [80]. We distinguish early postoperative hemorrhages occurring in the first 24 hours after surgery and late postoperative hemorrhages occurring beyond the first 24 hours postoperatively.

4.7.2. Prognosis

In our study, 18-month survival was 28%, locoregional recurrence was observed in 37% of cases with a mean delay of 170 days and the occurrence of distant metastases was observed in 37% of cases with a mean delay of 140 days.

Indeed, despite progress in the treatment of pancreatic cancers and new chemotherapy molecules, it remains today a cancer with a poor prognosis with a 5-year survival rate not exceeding 20% in patients who have had curative treatment [81,82].

Survival is even more reduced in patients whose tumor is unresectable with a median survival estimated at 4 months after diagnosis [83].

Recommendations and perspectives:

- The prognosis of pancreatic cancer remains dire. It is therefore necessary to increase scientific work to determine the histological factors such as tumor budding that may be involved in its aggressiveness in order to develop therapeutic strategies focused on these factors.
- The correlation between survival and tumor budding in pancreatic cancer has been demonstrated as is the case of our work through many studies. However, given its time-consuming, difficult and poorly reproducible analysis, BT remains little or not reported in histological reports. AI could facilitate this analysis, however, it is still an expensive technology that requires a profound restructuring of practices and priorities. In this context, the use of QUPATH software constitutes an advantageous alternative for pathologists in low-income countries which is equipped with many features for analyzing digitalized images on both HE and immunohistochemical or fluorescent staining. It also has the advantage

of being open to the update of new extensions that could considerably expand the field of analysis according to needs.

- The digitalization of microscopic slides or "virtual slides" is now part of the analysis in pathological anatomy. Beyond its educational contribution and in tele-expertise, it offers support for the development of AI analysis algorithms. It is to be hoped that the future generalization of the digitalization of slides and software will lead to controllable costs for all institutions.
- The use of artificial AI in the assessment of prognostic factors in pathological anatomy, in particular quantifiable scores such as BT, seems to offer better accuracy, reproducibility and speed of analysis. However, in order to definitively decide on its contribution compared to conventional morphological analysis, multicenter studies with a standardized approach are necessary. However, overall, in pathological anatomy, it is more reasonable to use AI always as a complement to human expertise rather than as a substitute, because an integrated assessment combining automated AI analysis and evaluation by pathologists can provide the best results.
- The use of AI software applied to pathological anatomy, however, finds its full interest in the evaluation of immunohistochemical scores in tumor pathology such as the assessment of the Ki67 proliferation index, particularly in neuroendocrine tumors, and the RO, RP and HER2 scores in breast cancer. Indeed, in current practice, the evaluation of these scores by morphological method is most often assessed in a semi-quantitative manner under the microscope. However, on AI software such as QUPATH, the pathologist could have a precise percentage of cell positivity, which contributes to considerably improving the risk stratification of certain tumors.

CONCLUSIONS

Pancreatic cancer is rare but remains serious with an overall 5-year survival rate, all stages combined, of around 7% to 8%.

On the anatomopathological level, pancreatic cancer is dominated by ductal adenocarcinoma which represents 90% of malignant tumors. The only curative treatment is oncological surgical resection. However, recurrence is reported in 70% of cases within 2 years.

Therefore, the anatomopathological examination is of capital importance in order to determine the histoprognostic factors predictive of tumor aggressiveness in order to adapt the therapeutic management. Among these histological factors, tumor budding has benefited as a new histoprognostic factor predictive of aggressiveness, recurrence and metastases in many solid cancers, particularly colon cancer. However, in pancreatic cancer, although most studies have demonstrated that tumor budding would also be an independent histoprognostic factor, this histological parameter is not yet systematically reported in anatomopathological reports.

It is in this context that our work is included, the objectives of which were to calculate the BT score in pancreatic adenocarcinomas by artificial intelligence and to analyze its prognostic value by correlation with clinical and histological parameters, overall survival and event-free survival.

This was a descriptive, cross-sectional study of cases of primary adenocarcinoma of the pancreas, collected from the pathological anatomy and cytology departments of the Internal Security Forces Hospital of La Marsa and the Charles Nicolle Hospital over a period of 14 years, between 2008-2022. We collected clinical, pathological and evolutionary data. The BT was evaluated by two approaches: a morphological approach which served as a basic reference and an approach on the QUPATH AI software. The morphological analysis was carried out on the HE-stained slides according to the recommendations established at the international BT consensus conference in 2016 for colon cancer. The digitalized approach was carried out after integration of the HE section images using the QUPATH artificial intelligence software applied to pathological anatomy.

Twenty-five patients were included in our study. The mean age was 62 ± 10 years with a male predominance (72%). Smoking was the predominant risk factor (56%). The most common clinical signs were deterioration of general condition (96%), abdominal pain (80%) and jaundice (72%). On the anatomopathological level the predominant histological subtype was conventional ductal carcinoma (85%), perineural sheaths were present in 80% of cases and vascular emboli were reported in 55% of cases.

In our study, BT was present in 100% of cases by morphological analysis and in 80% of cases by analysis on QUPATH software. These results, like those in the literature, suggest that tumor budding is a relatively frequent or even constant histological parameter in pancreatic cancer. This could explain on the one hand its aggressiveness and on the other hand could have a great diagnostic value of pancreatic cancer on biopsy samples.

In our study, high BT was found in 56% of cases by morphological method; it was 48% by QUPATH software. Similarly, the use of semi-automated analysis on QUPATH halved the number of Category BUD3 cases. These data suggest a reduction in false positives by using semi-automated analysis.

Thus, this approach using the QUPATH software seems more precise, objective, reproducible and has the advantage of allowing a reassessment of the BT at any time by other pathologists. However, in our study context, it should be remembered that the quality of the digitalized images is an essential requirement for the reliability of the results of BT analysis by artificial intelligence.

Overall, the difference observed in the assessment of tumor budding between the morphological approach and the QUPATH software approach was not statistically significant ($p = 0.589$). Therefore, this software could be an interesting, fast, accurate and freely accessible alternative for pathologists. This would contribute on the one hand to initiating artificial intelligence applied to pathological anatomy, particularly in our country, and on the other hand to facilitating the assessment of quantifiable histological criteria such as tumor budding in colon and pancreatic cancer but also prognostic immunohistochemical scores such as the Ki67 proliferation index and hormone receptors in other cancers.

However, overall, artificial intelligence applied to pathological anatomy is certainly advantageous, precise, objective and reproducible; it is however essential to always use it in addition to human morphological expertise which nevertheless constitutes a reliable reference base.

The analysis of the prognostic value of tumor budding in our study showed a statistically significant association between a high BT score and advanced age ($p=0.03$). Similarly, a high histological grade and a high BT significantly affected overall survival ($p=0.044$, $p=0.038$). These results, as well as those in the literature, provide additional evidence in favor of the poor prognostic value of tumor budding in pancreatic cancer. It is therefore necessary to start integrating it into the anatomopathological study now for a better risk stratification in patients with pancreatic cancer with a view to a more aggressive therapeutic strategy.

In this context, on the therapeutic level, if the presence of high tumor budding constitutes an indication for adjuvant chemotherapy in stage II colon cancer, this histological criterion seems, according to current recommendations, to have little impact on the decision for adjuvant chemotherapy in pancreatic cancer. However, it would have a predictive value for response to immunotherapy, which currently constitutes a promising therapy in pancreatic cancer.

In view of these results which reinforce the negative prognostic and potential therapeutic predictive value of tumor budding, it is necessary to increase scientific work on this subject, in particular to develop precise recommendations for the quantification of BT first morphologically and then on artificial intelligence software in order to integrate it into current practice for a better prognostic categorization of patients with pancreatic cancer.

REFERENCES

1. Hu JX, Zhao CF, Chen WB, Liu QC, Li QW, Lin YY, et al. Pancreatic cancer: a review of epidemiology, trends, and risk factors. World J Gastroenterol. 2021 Jul;27(27):4298-321.
2. Neuzillet C, Gaujoux S, Williet N, Bachet JB, Bauguion L, Colson Durand L, et al. Pancreatic cancer: French clinical practice guidelines for diagnosis, treatment and follow-up (SNFGE, FFCD, GERCOR, UNICANCER, SFCD, SFED, SFRO, ACHBT, AFC). Dig Liver Dis. 2018 Dec;50(12):1257-71.
3. Drouillard A, Manfredi S, Lepage C, Bouvier AM. Epidemiology of pancreatic cancer. Bull Cancer. Jan 2018;105(1):63-9.
4. Masiak Segit W, Rawicz Pruszyński K, Skórzewska M, Polkowski WP. Surgical treatment of pancreatic cancer. Pol Przegl Chir. 2018 Apr;90(2):45-53.
5. Petrova E, Zielinski V, Bolm L, Schreiber C, Knief J, Thorns C, et al. Tumor budding as a prognostic factor in pancreatic ductal adenocarcinoma. Virchows Arch. 2020 Apr;476(4):561-8.
6. Karamitopoulou E, Zlobec I, Born D, Kondi Pafiti A, Lykoudis P, Mellou A, et al. Tumor budding is a strong and independent prognostic factor in pancreatic cancer. Eur J Cancer. 2013 Mar;49(5):1032-9.
7. Chouat E, Zehani A, Chelly I, Njima M, Maghrebi H, Bani MA, et al. Tumor budding is a prognostic factor linked to epithelial mesenchymal transition in pancreatic ductal adenocarcinoma. Study report and literature review. Pancreatology. 2018 Jan;18(1):79-84.
8. Karamitopoulou E. Tumor budding cells, cancer stem cells and epithelial-mesenchymal transition-type cells in pancreatic cancer. Front Oncol. 2013 Jan;2:209.
9. Hase K, Shatney C, Johnson D, Trollope M, Vierra M. Prognostic value of tumor "budding" in patients with colorectal cancer. Say Colon Rectum. 1993 Jul;36(7):627-35.
10. Park SY, Choe G, Lee HS, Jung SY, Park JG, Kim WH. Tumor budding as an indicator of isolated tumor cells in lymph nodes from patients with node-negative colorectal cancer. Say Colon Rectum. 2005 Feb;48(2):292-302.
11. Lugli A, Kirsch R, Ajioka Y, Bosman F, Cathomas G, Dawson H, et al. Recommendations for reporting tumor budding in colorectal cancer based on the international tumor budding consensus conference (ITBCC) 2016. Mod Pathol. 2017 Sep;30(9):1299-311.
12. QuPath [Internet]. [accessed 15 June 2023]. Available at URL: https://qupath.github.io/.

13. Budau KL, Sigel CS, Bergmann L, Lüchtenborg AM, Wellner U, Schilling O, et al. Prognostic impact of tumor budding in intrahepatic cholangiocellular carcinoma. J Cancer. 2022 May;13(8):2457-71.
14. Crane CH, Varadhachary GR, Wolff RA, Fleming JB. Challenges in the study of adjuvant chemoradiation after pancreaticoduodenectomy. Ann Surg Oncol. 2010 Apr;17(4):950-2.
15. Thiery JP, Sleeman JP. Complex networks orchestrate epithelial-mesenchymal transitions. Nat Rev Mol Cell Biol. 2006 Feb;7(2):131-42.
16. Léger A. Artificial intelligence analysis of tumor budding and poorly differentiated clusters as new histoprognostic factors in non-metastatic colorectal cancer: literature review in 2021 [thesis: medicine]. Caen: University of Caen Normandy; 2021.
17. Wang LM, Kevans D, Mulcahy H, O'Sullivan J, Fennelly D, Hyland J, et al. Tumor budding is a strong and reproducible prognostic marker in T3N0 colorectal cancer. Am J Surg Pathol. 2009 Jan;33(1):134-41.
18. Karamitopoulou E, Zlobec I, Kölzer V, Kondi Pafiti A, Patsouris ES, Gennatas K, et al. Proposal for a 10-high-power-fields scoring method for the assessment of tumor budding in colorectal cancer. Mod Pathol. 2013 Feb;26(2):295-301.
19. Ishikawa Y, Akishima Fukasawa Y, Ito K, Akasaka Y, Yokoo T, Ishii T, et al. Histopathologic determinants of regional lymph node metastasis in early colorectal cancer. Cancer. 2008 Feb;112(4):924-33.
20. Nakamura T, Mitomi H, Kikuchi S, Ohtani Y, Sato K. Evaluation of the usefulness of tumor budding on the prediction of metastasis to the lung and liver after curative excision of colorectal cancer. Hepatogastroenterology. 2005 Sep;52(65):1432-5.
21. Ueno H, Mochizuki H, Hashiguchi Y, Hatsuse K, Fujimoto H, Hase K. Predictors of extrahepatic recurrence after resection of colorectal liver metastases. Br J Surg. 2004 Feb;91(3):327-33. Noel M, Fiscella K. Disparities in pancreatic cancer treatment and outcomes. Health Equity. 2019 Oct;3(1):532-40.
22. Horcic M, Koelzer VH, Karamitopoulou E, Terracciano L, Puppa G, Zlobec I, et al. Tumor budding score based on 10 high-power fields is a promising basis for a standardized prognostic scoring system in stage II colorectal cancer. Um Pathol. 2013 May;44(5):697-705. Billami W. Pancreatic cancer [thesis: medicine]. Tlemcen: Abou Bekr Belkaid University; 2015.
23. Sadozai H, Acharjee A, Gruber T, Gloor B, Karamitopoulou E. Pancreatic cancers with high grade tumor budding exhibit hallmarks of diminished anti-tumor immunity. Cancers. 2021 Mar;13(5):1090.

24. Hacking S, Nasim R, Lee L, Vitkovski T, Thomas R, Shaffer E, et al. Whole slide imaging and colorectal carcinoma: a validation study for tumor budding and stromal differentiation. Pathol Res Pract. 2020 Nov;216(11):153233.
25. Jepsen RK, Klarskov LL, Lippert MF, Novotny GW, Hansen TP, Christensen IJ, et al. Digital image analysis of pan-cytokeratin stained tumor slides for evaluation of tumor budding in pT1/pT2 colorectal cancer: results of a feasibility study. Pathol Res Pract. 2018 Sep;214(9):1273-81.
26. Weis CA, Kather JN, Melchers S, Al Ahmdi H, Pollheimer MJ, Langner C, et al. Automatic evaluation of tumor budding in immunohistochemically stained colorectal carcinomas and correlation to clinical outcome. Diagn Pathol. 2018 Aug;13(1):64.
27. Fauzi MA, Chen W, Knight D, Hampel H, Frankel WL, Gurcan MN. Tumor budding detection system in whole slide pathology images. J Med Syst. 2019 Dec;44(2):38.
28. Zhou T, Man Q, Li X, Xie Y, Hou X, Wang H, et al. Artificial intelligence-based comprehensive analysis of immune-stemness-tumor budding profile to predict survival of patients with pancreatic adenocarcinoma. Cancer Biol Med. 2023 Mar;20(3):196-217.
29. Bergler M, Benz M, Rauber D, Hartmann D, Kötter M, Eckstein M, et al. Automatic detection of tumor buds in pan-cytokeratin stained colorectal cancer sections by a hybrid image analysis approach. In: Reyes Aldasoro CC, Janowczyk A, Veta M, Bankhead P, Sirinukunwattana K, eds. Digital pathology. Cham: Springer; 2019. p. 83-90.
30. Caie PD, Turnbull AK, Farrington SM, Oniscu A, Harrison DJ. Quantification of tumor budding, lymphatic vessel density and invasion through image analysis in colorectal cancer. J Transl Med. 2014 Jun;12:156.
31. Pallua JD, Brunner A, Zelger B, Schirmer M, Haybaeck J. The future of pathology is digital. Pathol Res Pract. 2020 Sep;216(9):153040.
32. Bankhead P, Loughrey MB, Fernández JA, Dombrowski Y, McArt DG, Dunne PD, et al. QuPath: open source software for digital pathology image analysis. SciRep. 2017 Dec;7(1):16878.
33. Tanaka M, Yamauchi N, Ushiku T, Shibahara J, Hayashi A, Misumi K, et al. Tumor budding in intrahepatic cholangiocarcinoma: a predictor of postsurgery outcomes. Am J Surg Pathol. 2019 Sep;43(9):1180-90.
34. O'Connor K, Li Chang HH, Kalloger SE, Peixoto RD, Webber DL, Owen DA, et al. Tumor budding is an independent adverse prognostic factor in pancreatic ductal adenocarcinoma. Am J Surg Pathol. 2015 Apr;39(4):472-8.

35. Lohneis P, Sinn M, Klein F, Bischoff S, Striefler JK, Wislocka L, et al. Tumor buds determine prognosis in resected pancreatic ductal adenocarcinoma. Br J Cancer. 2018 May;118(11):1485-91.
36. Jiang H, Yang Y, Qian Y, Shao C, Lu J, Bian Y, et al. Tumor budding score is a strong and independent prognostic factor in patients with pancreatic ductal adenocarcinoma: an evaluation of whole slide pathology images of large sections. Front Oncol. 2021 Nov;11:740212.
37. Lawlor RT, Veronese N, Nottegar A, Malleo G, Smith L, Demurtas J, et al. Prognostic Role of High-Grade Tumor Budding in Pancreatic Ductal Adenocarcinoma: A Systematic Review and Meta-Analysis with a Focus on Epithelial to Mesenchymal Transition. Cancers. 2019 Jan 19;11(1):113.
38. Chen S, Zhang N, Jiang L, Gao F, Shao J, Wang T, et al. Clinical use of a machine learning histopathological image signature in diagnosis and survival prediction of clear cell renal cell carcinoma. Int J Cancer. 2021 Feb;148(3):780-90.
39. Tabata K, Mori I, Sasaki T, Itoh T, Shiraishi T, Yoshimi N, et al. Whole-slide imaging at primary pathological diagnosis: validation of whole-slide imaging-based primary pathological diagnosis at twelve Japanese academic institutes. Pathol Int. 2017 Nov;67(11):547-54.
40. Loughrey MB, Kelly PJ, Houghton OP, Coleman HG, Houghton JP, Carson A, et al. Digital slide viewing for primary reporting in gastrointestinal pathology: a validation study. Virchows Arch. 2015 Aug;467(2):137-44.
41. ESMO 2021 - A new independent prognostic factor in stage III colon cancer: tumor budding [Internet]. 2021 [accessed 15 September 2023]. Available at: https://www.aphp.fr/contenu/esmo-2021-un-nouveau-facteur-pronostique-independant-dans-les-cancers-coliques-de-stade-iii.
42. Zlobec I, Berger MD, Lugli A. Tumor budding and its clinical implications in gastrointestinal cancers. Br J Cancer. 2020 Sep;123(5):700-8.
43. Neoptolemos JP, Palmer DH, Ghaneh P, Psarelli EE, Valle JW, Halloran CM, et al. Comparison of adjuvant gemcitabine and capecitabine with gemcitabine monotherapy in patients with resected pancreatic cancer (ESPAC-4): a multicenter, open-label, randomized, phase 3 trial. Lancet. 2017 Mar 11;389(10073):1011-24.
44. Lohneis P, Sinn M, Klein F, Bischoff S, Striefler JK, Wislocka L, et al. Tumor buds determine prognosis in resected pancreatic ductal adenocarcinoma. Br J Cancer. 2018 May 29;118(11):1485-91.

45. Terry S, Savagner P, Ortiz-Cuaran S, Mahjoubi L, Saintigny P, Thiery JP, et al. New insights into the role of EMT in tumor immune escape. Mol Oncol. 2017 Jul;11(7):824-46.
46. Sadozai H, Acharjee A, Gruber T, Gloor B, Karamitopoulou E. Pancreatic Cancers with High Grade Tumor Budding Exhibit Hallmarks of Diminished Anti-Tumor Immunity. Cancers. 2021 Mar 4;13(5):1090.
47. De Oliveira ML, Winter JM, Schafer M, Cunningham SC, Cameron JL, Yeo CJ, et al. Assessment of complications after pancreatic surgery: a novel grading system applied to 633 patients undergoing pancreaticoduodenectomy. Ann Surg. 2006 Dec;244(6):931-7.
48. Sohn TA, Yeo CJ, Cameron JL, Koniaris L, Kaushal S, Abrams RA, et al. Resected adenocarcinoma of the pancreas-616 patients: results, outcomes, and prognostic indicators. J Gastrointest Surg. 2000 Nov;4(6):567-79.
49. Pannegeon V, Pessaux P, Sauvanet A, Vullierme MP, Kianmanesh R, Belghiti J. Pancreatic fistula after distal pancreatectomy: predictive risk factors and value of conservative treatment. Arch Surg. 2006 Nov;141(11):1071-6.
50. Petermann D, Ksontini R, Halkic N, Demartines N. Cephalic pancreatudoodenomectomy: indications, results and management of complications. Rev Med Suisse. 2008 Jun;163(25):1563-6.
51. Kimura W. Surgical anatomy of the pancreas for limited resection. J Hepatobiliary Pancreat Surg. 2000 May;7(5):473-9.
52. Ahmad NA, Lewis JD, Ginsberg GG, Haller DG, Morris JB, Williams NN, et al. Long term survival after pancreatic resection for pancreatic adenocarcinoma. Am J Gastroenterol. 2001 Sep;96(9):2609-15.
53. Ferrone CR, Brennan MF, Gonen M, Coit DG, Fong Y, Chung S, et al. Pancreatic adenocarcinoma: the actual 5-year survivors. J Gastrointest Surg. 2008 Apr;12(4):701-6.
54. Fouquet T. Risk factors for early recurrence after cephalic pancreatudoodenomectomy for ductal adenocarcinoma of the head of the pancreas. About 166 patients [thesis: medicine]. Nancy. Henri Poincaré University; 2011.
55. Nagtegaal ID, Odze RD, Klimstra D, Paradis V, Rugge M, Schirmacher P, et al. The 2019 WHO classification of tumors of the digestive system. Histopathology. 2020 Jan;76(2):182-8.

56. Schlitter AM, Segler A, Steiger K, Michalski CW, Jäger C, Konukiewitz B, et al. Molecular, morphological and survival analysis of 177 resected pancreatic ductal adenocarcinomas (PDACs): identification of prognostic subtypes. SciRep. 2017 Feb;7:41064.
57. Haeberle L, Esposito I. Pathology of pancreatic cancer. Transl Gastroenterol Hepatol. 2019 Jun;4:50.
58. Esposito I, Penzel R, Chaib Harrireche M, Barcena U, Bergmann F, Riedl S, et al. Tenascin C and annexin II expression in the process of pancreatic carcinogenesis. J Pathol. 2006 Apr;208(5):673-85.
59. Liang D, Shi S, Xu J, Zhang B, Qin Y, Ji S, et al. New insights into perineural invasion of pancreatic cancer: more than pain. Biochim Biophys Acta. 2016 Apr;1865(2):111-22.
60. Versteijne E, Suker M, Groothuis K, Akkermans Vogelaar JM, Besselink MG, Bonsing BA, et al. Preoperative chemoradiotherapy versus immediate surgery for resectable and borderline resectable pancreatic cancer: results of the Dutch randomized phase III PREOPANC trial. J Clin Oncol. 2020 Jun;38(16):1763-73.
61. Chatterjee D, Katz MH, Rashid A, Wang H, Iuga AC, Varadhachary GR, et al. Perineural and intraneural invasion in posttherapy pancreaticoduodenectomy specimens predicts poor prognosis in patients with pancreatic ductal adenocarcinoma. Am J Surg Pathol. 2012 Mar;36(3):409-17.
62. Liang D, Shi S, Xu J, Zhang B, Qin Y, Ji S, et al. New insights into perineural invasion of pancreatic cancer: more than pain. Biochim Biophys Acta. 2016 Apr;1865(2):111-22.
63. Takahashi C, Shridhar R, Huston J, Meredith K. Correlation of tumor size and survival in pancreatic cancer. J Gastrointest Oncol. 2018 Oct;9(5):910-21.
64. Gnerlich JL, Luka SR, Deshpande AD, Dubray BJ, Weir JS, Carpenter DH, et al. Microscopic margins and patterns of treatment failure in resected pancreatic adenocarcinoma. Arch Surg. 2012 Aug;147(8):753-60.
65. Ministry of Health. Cancer Registry Data 2010-2014. [Online]. Mar 2021 [Accessed 24 Oct 2023]; [157 pages]. Available at: https://www.institutsalahazaiez.com/medias/bulletin%202010_2014_final%20(1).pdf

66. Iodice S, Gandini S, Maisonneuve P, Lowenfels AB. Tobacco and the risk of pancreatic cancer: a review and meta-analysis. Langenbecks Arch Surg. 2008 Jul;393(4):535-45.
67. Bosetti C, Lucenteforte E, Silverman DT, Petersen G, Bracci PM, Ji BT, et al. Cigarette smoking and pancreatic cancer: an analysis from the international pancreatic cancer case-control consortium (Panc4). Ann Oncol. 2012 Jul;23(7):1880-8.
68. Tramacere I, Scotti L, Jenab M, Bagnardi V, Bellocco R, Rota M, et al. Alcohol drinking and pancreatic cancer risk: a meta-analysis of the dose-risk relationship. Int J Cancer. 2010 Mar;126(6):1474-86.
69. Rawla P, Sunkara T, Gaduputi V. Epidemiology of pancreatic cancer: global trends, etiology and risk factors. World J Oncol. 2019 Feb;10(1):10-27.
70. Le Cosquer G, Maulat C, Bournet B, Cordelier P, Buscail E, Buscail L. Pancreatic cancer in chronic pancreatitis: pathogenesis and diagnostic approach. Cancers. 2023 Jan;15(3):761.
71. Tchuisse Noukoua C, Duran U, Mutijima E, Noumessi PM, Nchimi A. Cancers of the exocrine pancreas. EMC – Hepatology 2020;35(4):1-14 [Article 7-106-A-12]
72. Wood LD, Canto MI, Jaffee EM, Simeone DM. Pancreatic cancer: pathogenesis, screening, diagnosis, and treatment. Gastroenterology. 2022 Aug;163(2):386-402.
73. Noel M, Fiscella K. Disparities in pancreatic cancer treatment and outcomes. Health Equity. 2019 Oct;3(1):532-40.
74. Zhao Z, Liu W. Pancreatic cancer: a review of risk factors, diagnosis, and treatment. Technol Cancer Res Treat. 2020 Jan;19:1533033820962117.
75. Billami W. Pancreatic cancer [thesis: medicine]. Tlemcen: Abou Bekr Belkaid University; 2015.
76. Perik TH, Van Genugten EJ, Aarntzen EG, Smit EJ, Huisman HJ, Hermans JJ. Quantitative CT perfusion imaging in patients with pancreatic cancer: a systematic review. Abdom Radiol. 2022 Sep;47(9):3101-17.
77. Yang J, Xu R, Wang C, Qiu J, Ren B, You L. Early screening and diagnosis strategies of pancreatic cancer: a comprehensive review. Common Cancer. 2021 Dec;41(12):1257-74.
78. Isaji S, Mizuno S, Windsor JA, Bassi C, Fernández Del Castillo C, Hackert T, et al. International consensus on definition and criteria of borderline resectable pancreatic ductal adenocarcinoma 2017. Pancreatology. 2018 Jan;18(1):2-11.

79. Yin T, Qin T, Wei K, Shen M, Zhang Z, Wen J, et al. Comparison of safety and effectiveness between laparoscopic and open pancreatoduodenectomy: a systematic review and meta-analysis. Int J Surg. 2022 Sep;105:106799.
80. Van Der Gaag NA, Rauws EJ, Van Eijck CJ, Bruno MJ, Van Der Harst E, Kubben FM, et al. Preoperative biliary drainage for cancer of the head of the pancreas. N Engl J Med. 2010 Jan;362(2):129-37.
81. Okusaka T, Furuse J. Recent advances in chemotherapy for pancreatic cancer: evidence from Japan and recommendations in guidelines. J Gastroenterol. 2020 Apr;55(4):369-82.
82. Dusch N, Lietzmann A, Barthels F, Niedergethmann M, Rückert F, Wilhelm TJ. International study group of pancreatic surgery definitions for postpancreatectomy complications: applicability at a high-volume center. Scand J Surg. 2017 Sep;106(3):216-23.
83. Birkmeyer JD, Stukel TA, Siewers AE, Goodney PP, Wennberg DE, Lucas FL. Surgeon volume and operative mortality in the United States. N Engl J Med. 2003 Nov;349(22):2117-27 .

ANNEXES

Annex 1: WHO classification of pancreatic carcinomas 2019 (40)

Ductal adenocarcinoma unspecified

Colloid carcinoma

Poorly cohesive carcinoma

Signet ring cell carcinoma

Unspecified medullary carcinoma

Adenosquamous carcinoma

Hepatoid carcinoma

Large cell carcinoma with rhabdoid phenotype

Undifferentiated carcinoma, unspecified

Undifferentiated carcinoma with osteoclast-like giant cells

Acinar cell carcinoma

Acinar cell cystadenocarcinoma

Mixed acinoneuroendocrine carcinoma

Mixed acinar-endocrine-ductal carcinoma

Mixed acinar-ductal carcinoma

Pancreatoblastoma

Solid pseudopapillary neoplasm of the pancreas

Solid pseudopapillary neoplasm with high-grade carcinoma

Appendix 2: National Comprehensive Cancer Network (NCCN) resectability criteria (11)

	Resectable tumor	Borderline Tumor	Unresectable tumor
Portal vein Superior mesenteric vein	Preservation of the fatty interface	Contact, deformation or occlusion with anatomical conformation allowing consideration of vascular reconstruction	Contact, deformation or occlusion without possible vascular reconstruction
Superior mesenteric artery	Preservation of the fatty interface	Tumor contact less than 180° from the circumference	Tumor contact greater than 180° of the circumference
Gastroduodenal artery Hepatic artery	Preservation of the fatty interface	Involvement up to the hepatic artery in a short segment without extension to the celiac trunk	Long-term involvement or extension to the celiac trunk
Celiac trunk Aorta Inferior vena cava	Preservation of the fatty interface	Preservation of the fatty interface	Vascular damage
Others			N2 adenopathies metastases

Appendix 3: AJCC TNM classification in its 8th edition of 2017

T1: Size less than or equal to 2 cm

T1a: Size less than or equal to 0.5 cm

T1b: Size strictly greater than 0.5cm and strictly less than 1cm

T1c: Size greater than or equal to 1 cm and less than or equal to 2 cm

T2: Size strictly greater than 2 cm and less than or equal to 4 cm
T3: Size strictly greater than 4 cm N0: no lymph nodes affected N1: 1 to 3 lymph nodes affected

N2: 4 or more affected lymph nodes

M0: No metastases

M1: Presence of metastases

INTEREST OF THE STUDY OF TUMOR BUDDING IN PRIMITIVE ADENOCARCINOMA OF THE PANCREAS: ANALYSIS ON DIGITAL IMAGES

Summary

Introduction :

Tumor budding (TB) has been identified as a new prognostic factor in many cancers, particularly pancreatic cancer. The objectives of our work were to calculate the TB score by artificial intelligence and to analyze its prognostic value by correlation with clinical and histological parameters, overall survival and event-free survival.

Methods:

This was a descriptive, cross-sectional, bicentric study of pancreatic adenocarcinoma cases from 2008 to 2022. We assessed BT by two methods: morphological and QUPATH software. Two groups were identified: low (BUD1) and high (BUD2, BUD3). We compared the results of the two analysis methods and determined the association of BT with clinical, histological, overall survival and event-free survival factors.

Results :

Twenty-five cases were included in the study. The mean age of the patients was 62 ± 10 years with a male predominance of 72%. BT was present in 100% of cases by morphological analysis and in 80% of cases using the digitalized approach on QUPATH. A high BT score was found in 56% of cases by morphological method; it was 48% by the QUPATH software. BT was category BUD3 in 36% by morphological method versus 12% by semi-automated analysis. The comparative analysis of the two methods did not show any statistically significant difference (p = 0.589). Furthermore, a statistically significant association was observed between a high BT score and advanced age (p = 0.03). No significant link was found with other clinical parameters. Regarding the survival study, high BT had a notable impact on overall survival with a statistically significant difference (p=0.038).

Conclusion :

BT is an additional prognostic factor in pancreatic cancer. QUPATH software could be a promising and accessible tool for pathologists to assess TB and integrate it into their pathology reports.

Keywords: Carcinoma, Pancreas, Tumor budding, Prognosis, Artificial intelligence

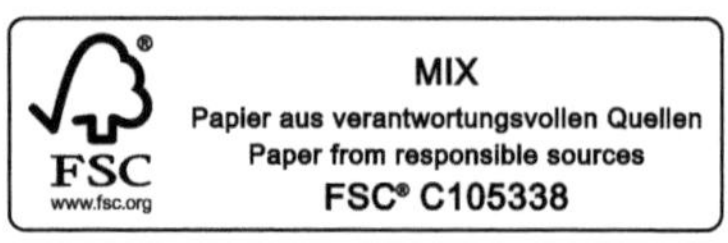

Printed by Books on Demand GmbH, Norderstedt / Germany